DRESSING ON THE SIDE

(and Other Diet Myths Debunked)

DRESSING ON THE SIDE

(and Other Diet Myths Debunked)

11 Science-Based Ways to Eat More, Stress Less, and Feel Great About Your Body

JACLYN LONDON, MS, RD, CDN

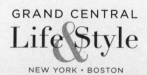

GRAND CENTRAL
Life & Style
NEW YORK · BOSTON

Grand Central Life & Style
Hachette Book Group
1290 Avenue of the Americas, New York, NY 10104
grandcentrallifeandstyle.com
twitter.com/grandcentralpub

First Edition: January 2019

Grand Central Life & Style is an imprint of Grand Central Publishing. The Grand Central Life & Style name and logo are trademarks of Hachette Book Group, Inc.

The publisher is not responsible for websites (or their content) that are not owned by the publisher.

The Hachette Speakers Bureau provides a wide range of authors for speaking events. To find out more, go to www.hachettespeakersbureau.com or call (866) 376-6591.

Library of Congress Control Number: 2018952143

ISBNs: 978-1-5387-4745-2 (hardcover), 978-1-5387-4747-6 (ebook)

Printed in the United States of America

LSC-H

10 9 8 7 6 5 4 3 2 1

*For my best friends—the bravest,
most compassionate, and most inspiring
superheroes on the planet: I love you,
Mom and Dad.*

Contents

1

Ugh...I Need a Detox

This chapter will help you...

- understand some real information about the human metabolism;
- swap toxic diet "language" for happier, healthier terminology; and
- tell the difference between a fad diet and nutrition information you can *actually use*.

Picture This:

It's January 1, and your head feels like it's going to explode. For the last five weeks, you've been hungover (okay, maybe since football season, as long as we're starting the year off from a *place of honesty*, and all...).

You're hangry; your head aches; your eyes are puffy; your face is puffy; hell, your right toenail looks a little bloated. You have to make resolutions, clean up your living space, invest in your kids' college fund (regardless of whether you even *have* children), remodel and refinance your home, and make amends with anyone you've ever alienated or by whom you've felt rejected. Plus, you *need* to start meditating (like, *at least twice a day...maybe you need some crystals, too?*), and on top of all of this: *You have to go to work tomorrow.*

(The world is so *cruel!*)

Once you've managed to hoist yourself out of bed and officially raise the blinds on the New Year, you think to yourself, *This is the year I'm going to lose weight.* But *how?* You've already been on *all the diets.* Right? I mean, who hasn't tried a low-carb breakfast and a vegan lunch?

Okay, think, you say to yourself. *Who would know how and where to start?* And out of nowhere, your phone rings: It's your mom. She's starting the Whole30 diet *today*, and it's *so amazing*! She lost five pounds in the last *hour* since she started it. *Must be all of that chopping and meal prepping,* you think.

Once you finally pry her off the phone, you log in to Facebook. Cousin Joe has gone seventeen hours ("and counting!") on his new fast (yes, he's not eating for twenty-four hours, and there isn't any actual religious reason or promised spiritual ascension for doing so). His latest status says he's "bio-hacking," which you have to reread a few times because it sounds like some form of cyberterrorism (*Wait, can he see me through this little camera on my screen?! OMG*), but it's actually just Silicon Valley–speak for "dieting."

(He's gotten so disciplined since he moved to Marin!)

Your favorite blogger? She's eating apples for a week. Nothing else. *Just apples.* Is this real? Apparently, it's not only real, but it's #clean #healthy #vegan.

Later, you call your dad to check in and wish him a happy New Year, and he tells you: "Went to the doc this morning; he says I need to be on a 'low sodium diet,' so I threw away all the saltshakers in the house. Uncle Jim's doing it with me—we're going out for Chinese tonight!"

Weird, you think to yourself. Your favorite cuff bracelet could barely squeeze onto your pinky finger the last time you dipped a dumpling into soy sauce, but maybe that was because you're *allergic* to soy? *I should try a detox,* you think. It sounds very clean, wholesome, *transcendent*, even. "Detox" sounds like something the super-jacked VP at work does after his mornings at CrossFit and before his "Clean-Mean-Green-2B-LEAN" protein shake, or what the yoga-*obsessed* twenty-three-year-old *retired* model you met at your nephew's daycare does after too many sips of organic vodka.

It sounds like the type of thing that only someone who wants to be "*the BEST version of myself this year!*" would do while uploading *to Instagram* from a silent meditation retreat in the desert. #cactusselfie #newyearnewme.

(I wonder if phones are even allowed on silent retreats? you wonder aloud to your houseplant.)

I should try it; if there's anyone who needs to detox right now, it's me.

And just like that, you boil a pot of hot water to sip (*with lemon, of course! I mean, you're starting RIGHT NOW!! And what else is even safe any-more?!)* and take a seat at your computer.

You open Google, type in "detox diet," and leap—"clear heart, open mind!"—into the land of diet claims, cleanses, kale, quinoa, and a *ton* of *confusion.*

"Why Am I So Confused???" Nutrition Research 101

Here's a secret I'm going to let you in on *right now* (you may already know this, given that you're reading this book): Detoxes are bullsh*t. Actually, they're a lot more than that: Detoxification, in general, is a real thing—both metabolically speaking and as part of a behavior change interven-tion in the beginning stage of addiction therapy treatment. The idea of "detoxing" is being used incorrectly by the diet/wellness world. Periods of extreme eating (or *drinking*) do not expedite the functions your liver already performs—all day, every day. As long as you're alive and have functioning vital organs while reading this book, you're *detoxing right now!* Extolling the benefits of liver "detoxes" is like being impressed by seeing a painter painting or a pilot flying (*it's cool, but part of the job description!*). So consider this my memo to all forms of media, everywhere: "Attention, media: Stop telling my vital organs how to do their job! They know what they're doing, and they're doing just great, thanks! They're the hardest-working organs I know!"

So how did all things health, weight, and feeling good about yourself get so damn complicated? Part of the reason that weight loss seems out of reach is because there's so much conflicting information out there. Another problematic reason why we're so profoundly confused about what to eat? Science is hard! And on top of that, it's often even harder to communicate. Translating scientific data into a tangible, relatable, and prescriptive plan of action for better health and weight loss is made even more challenging by the fact that nutrition science is evolving constantly. Therefore, how to *actually use* evidence to develop public health recommendations is detached from its very real, very nuanced applications to the realities of our everyday lives.

My concern with many "detoxes," fad diets, or health programs is that *seemingly* big results are coming out of small-scale studies with very few participants and with *very* short durations. These studies don't have much in the way of statistical power, yet they do often make headlines. That's for a few reasons, but it's predominantly because of the way we consume content and information these days. It's exciting (to a network or website) when an idea that's previously been well established, or commonly believed to be true—like, say, the concept of "low-fat diets"—is *disrupted* by the idea of something else—like, say, that *coconut oil will solve all your problems.* (For those just tuning in to the trend right now: Coconut oil is a plant-based, mostly saturated fat that packs 14 grams (g) of fat per tablespoon—12 grams of which is saturated.)

Another issue is that in nutrition research, *association* is not the same thing as causation—and that's a major problem when it comes to understanding how the science of a diet, eating philosophy, or weight-management program actually *works.*

Here's the difference: *Association* is a term that researchers and health-care professionals use to show links based on statistical analysis in a population or *cohort* study. These range in sample size, but the big ones in nutrition include some you may have heard of (and even participated in!), such as the Nurses' Health Studies and the National Health and Nutrition Examination Surveys. It's from these long-term analyses of population that we gain insight into what people eat, how much they eat, when they eat, and how their weight (and plenty of other measurable health indicators, like blood panels, blood pressure, and metabolic indicators) is affected by the foods they eat frequently. When population studies give us associative results, they're generated by running data through statistical analyses and finding links among them. Some results of recent population health studies you may have heard about already:

- Diets low in fiber and high in processed foods are linked to a higher risk of developing lifestyle-related cancers.
- Diets high in saturated fat, added sugar, and sodium are associated with cardiovascular disease.
- Diets high in vegetables and fruit are associated with a longer life span.

When you hear about causative data in the news, it's typically in conjunction with FDA approval of a new drug, a comparison of two different diet types, or a comparison of a dietary supplement to a placebo (in which the supplement would have to demonstrate a degree of safety to be used with human subjects altogether). Trials compare groups of individuals and are at their strongest statistical power when they're blind (*double-blind* means neither the subjects nor the researchers know who's in which group; *single-blind* means the researchers know who's doing *what*, but participants do not).

Some examples of causation-determining studies that probably sound familiar to you:

- Low-fat diets are more effective for weight loss than low-carb diets.
- Low-carb diets are more effective for weight loss than low-fat diets.
- Athletes who drink a high-carb supplement versus a placebo drink before a marathon run faster than the control group.

In pharmacological studies, researchers look at hard data outcomes in population sets for whom they think a drug could be beneficial after (often) short-duration trials. A good example is the testing of blood sugar–lowering medications (also called *oral hypoglycemic agents*) in people with prediabetes. Once the data show that a medication works for its intended purpose (side effects are evaluated for safety, too), the trial ends, the study is published, and a drug is often approved by the FDA for prescription-based use among a specific population set.

When studies are reported, the part of any outcome deemed worthy of mainstream consumer interest is the part that shares the very basic bottom line of the study's findings—*not* the fact that the data looked at only seventeen people, or that all participants were on weight-loss diets, or that there was an *Abs of Steel* video workout requirement (*you get the picture, right?!*). A good story is a good story, but it often leaves out the really important nuances, details, and warnings that would allow people to understand what the findings were actually based on and for whom the treatment is recommended (or *not* recommended!).

To be clear, this book is *not* a diatribe against using science to drive news or boost "clicks." But it's crucial to remember that not all science you hear about day-to-day is created equal. And since not all of us are scientists, it's pretty tough to actually *know* what's well-established scientific consensus versus what's controversial or new.

Another mistake we make when hearing about and looking into scientific data is that we take pieces of the data and form a theory about it that sounds just peachy. If *that*, then *this*, right? But it's not that simple. Case in point: the word *detox* as it relates to nutrition and biology. (*Full circle!*)

WHAT'S THE DIFFERENCE BETWEEN "DETOX" AND "ELIMINATION"?

Elimination is another buzzword that's overused yet poorly understood by most of us. Elimination diets are often very useful—but not for the reasons the internet has led you to believe. An elimination diet is the process of removing common allergens from what you eat and drink every day, and slowly adding them, one by one, back into your diet so that you can determine exactly *what type of food—or specific nutrient within said food*—is causing you discomfort. Biochemically speaking, an elimination diet is a way to identify specific triggers to your body's immune response that make you feel sick, or specific foods that simply don't agree with you and make you uncomfortable. Elimination diets are often an investigative tool that medical professionals—including gastroenterologists, allergists, immunologists, and dietitians—use to help them (and *you*) diagnose an allergy or intolerance, a process that can take anywhere from days to weeks to *months*! But elimination diets for weight loss? Sure, you might lose some weight at first—especially if you've cut out breaded, deep-fried mozzarella sticks to determine if you're lactose-intolerant or gluten-sensitive. But any weight loss would occur because of the *types of foods* you've eliminated during this process, *not* because there's a chemical compound naturally found in food (in this case, *lactose* or *gluten*) that has made you pack on the pounds! When we miss this small but absolutely *crucial* distinction—well, that's when we get ourselves into hot water with weight loss and evade what's ultimately our real goal: weight loss that's *permanent* (i.e., successful weight loss that eventually turns into *weight maintenance* over time).

Research has shown that periods of repeated restriction continuously beget weight-cycling and diet-dependence—a process in which we obsess about our diets, watch as our weight fluctuates consistently and dramatically up and down more than 10 percent, and completely upend everything we thought we knew about eating for both health and happiness. Diet-dependence is, in its own way, an addictive (and potentially destructive) habit: At first, on *any* diet, we lose weight as we restrict the amount of food (aka calories) we eat. Over time, the more we lose, the slower our metabolic rate, which makes it that much harder to lose *any more weight*. If we keep eating the same amount as we did when we started? Well, then we start gaining it back, a process that's psychologically anxiety-provoking at *best*, and metabolically and *psychologically* damaging at worst! The more we do this—yo-yo dieting—the more our metabolism grows confused and exhausted and just wants to be left the hell *alone*. Which only makes it increasingly difficult over time to lose and maintain weight. Not only is the yo-yo dieting population more likely to suffer from depression, but they're also more likely to stay overweight and *gain* weight instead of losing weight in the long-term.

The more you yo-yo, the more likely it is that your little yo-yo string will wear out. In humans, that can result in weight gain, insulin-resistance, and metabolic syndrome.

#protip

Where *do* you need to cold-turkey detox? From the idea that in order to make a real change in your life—that is, lose a few pounds—you have to do something extremely difficult, endure being extremely overwhelmed, and commit to a completely impossible plan that you can barely tolerate for a few weeks, only to gain it all right back when you sniff at a slice of pizza. Real change is best served with a strategy—a game plan for actions that prioritize you, your short- and long-term health, and how you feel about your body in ways that meet the demands of your schedule and personal time.

So think of this book as ground zero for weight loss. To make substantial, lasting change that satisfies you mentally, emotionally, and physically, we have to detox your painful dieting experiences, confused ideologies, and the multitude of mixed messages floating around in your already-jam-packed brain, and start with some weight-loss basics: Real weight loss has to feel relatable and attainable, and the changes you make need to be (they *have to be!*) seamless enough to fit into your everyday lifestyle. If the necessary changes challenge you beyond your inner and outer expectations of yourself, you'll fail. If they're so "easy" that you're not changing in the slightest? They won't work, either. Think of it using a Pareto principle (*you've likely heard of this used in other ways before, right?*): an 80:20 rule. The changes you make through this book and beyond will be integrated into your lifestyle. They'll be 80 percent shifts that meet your current schedule, adaptability and willingness to change, and current lifestyle. And they'll be 20 percent aspirational—challenging but inspiring enough to make you want to push yourself to try slightly new things, one step at a time.

We need to detox from this diet-culture-induced *wellness* mindset, starting with some honesty about what our personal goals actually *are*. We need to feel empowered, we need to get our information from the appropriate sources, and we need to inspire in ourselves the types of behavior with which we feel appropriately comfortable and mildly challenged.

Yep, you're about to eat, sleep, and breathe this ratio!

EVERYBODY'S DOING IT, RIGHT?

If you feel like everyone you know is extolling the virtues of *this* detox or *that* cleanse, it can be even harder to struggle with following the rules or with the realization that you're not having the same success. But what's important to remember is that we all have a tendency to generalize things that work for us. If one person is able to say, "OMG, I lost so much weight cutting out carbs!," for someone else that might mean: "I tried to live on meat and butter and cheese, and all I got were four extra pounds and a *gallstone*!" (*Ouch! Hang in there, buddy!*)

It's hard to evaluate a diet and readily determine what will work for a specific type of person. But to be fair, we *are* getting better at this! Now we're seeing different types of diets tested on people with certain similarities in their gut microbiome (DNA you find in the cells of your intestinal wall) that can help get us even more specific in terms of who should be on what type of diet for a certain type of disease prevention, or what makes some versus others at risk for obesity.

Since nutrition research takes place in both population studies with large cohorts (these look at patterns and search for links between food and health to know more about positives and negatives, and what to study *next* in more detail) *and* randomized controlled trials (where there's an intervention to see if there's a positive effect in one group versus another), we're always relying on *links* to inform us concerning what works versus what doesn't—not *actual, hard data*.

If it's that hard to test, then how did the fad diet world get to be so powerful? Well, in addition to what I talked about earlier, I think that part of it is that fad diets can seem more exciting than simply adopting good habits. But I also think it's because fad diets come with a set number of rules, and because it often seems a lot easier to follow an amazing-looking person's long list of rules than it is to make balanced, nutritious choices that keep the taste of things you like while allowing some room both for you to have *fun* with what you eat and to challenge you to choose things just *slightly* adjacent to your comfort zone (for some of you, that's matcha; for others, it's foraging in Brazil for the next *açaí*! And for others still, it's eating vegetables and potatoes and spinach—but without the half gallon of heavy cream). It's also because when we see a biological plausibility that something could affect you in a certain way, there's a degree of excitement surrounding the topic itself.

Notice what we *don't* say here? "Everything in moderation." *Moderation* is so outrageously subjective that it's lost all semblance of meaning. Seriously, this is a pop quiz: Try to define the term *moderation* as it applies to eating food. Compare with your neighbor. See how those definitions differ? If two people can't agree, what makes so many of us believe that using the term *moderation* has a meaningful impact on the masses? Quite the opposite. In fact, moderation is too vague, too intangible to put to use—so it just becomes a platitude rather than an action plan. (*It's a bit like the trope "work–life balance," as it relates to what you eat, no?!*)

We like things that are tangible and quantifiable, and to that end, elimination diets give us satisfaction—but moderation fuels diets; it does *not* quell them.

The truth is, there is one category of food in which we can all go *nuts*, and that's produce. You got it: veggies and fruit. But it's not quite as sexy to say, "Hit that cucumber hard!" (although I guess it *is*, in some circles...) as it is to say, "Eat all the bacon you want!" More on that later.

Rebranding "Detox" as "Biology"

Where did that concept of detoxing as a means to a "wellness" end come from? And if it's *totally* wrong, why is it seemingly everywhere?!

Well, *lots* of reasons, but I have a few thoughts on how this went from a sexy-sounding word to a full-blown search engine optimization (SEO) term. A lot of it has to do with very smart marketing on the very important work your body's organs already do—and leads us *humans* to naturally think we can help them to do *better*.

What *detoxification* actually refers to is the combined processes of human digestion, absorption, and metabolism. In other words, "detox" is undergoing a *rebrand* when it comes to its reference in your everyday life; we can call it *basic human BIOLOGY*!

Digestion begins in the mouth—it's the first "organ" of the digestive tract when we really think about it. When we chew, we begin to digest and absorb certain nutrients, and that process continues all the way down the esophagus and into the stomach, where it continues. The small intestine is where the real *magic* starts happening. Our intestines are designed to absorb what we *need*—macronutrients (protein, fat, carbs) and micronutrients (essential vitamins and minerals)—into the bloodstream and to excrete much of what we don't need—including what could potentially be harmful to us—via the rest of the GI tract (the large intestine, colon, and rectum) in fecal form. (*PS, isn't that such a refined way of saying "poop"?!*)

What the GI tract misses in terms of potential "toxins" may be absorbed into the bloodstream and then metabolized by the liver, also known as the "powerhouse" of the body. Blood carries nutrients that we've consumed in *excess of what we personally need* (anything from fat to potassium to vitamin B_3—you name it!) away from the GI tract and into the liver to be further broken down into substances the body can use (nontoxic/necessary medications, for example) or into smaller, more user-friendly forms for the *rest* of the body to use more efficiently (like when we eat Thanksgiving turkey, aka protein, and our bodies break it down into amino acids, including the sleep-promoting tryptophan).

The liver does basically *everything* we could ever want for our bodies in terms of *cleansing*—in fact, it does much more than a sensible "cleansing"; it deep-cleans and sanitizes everything going in and repackages it into something brand-new (and much more useful). The liver will break down and filter what it can use and eliminate what it *can't* use via the intestine or the bloodstream.

The liver takes what's left over and uses it to make bile out of the by-products of the compounds formerly known as *toxins* (basically anything consumed in surplus of what the body can use or store at a given moment, like water and cholesterol).

Bile is a substance made up of what's essentially metabolic waste—cholesterol, water, certain types of fat, and bile salts—that serves as an emulsifying agent to help us digest and absorb the nutrients in our food. What's no longer useful for the body (excess of the good stuff, or stuff we accidentally ate, like a random fruit fly or a swallowed piece of gum) will be eliminated through the bowel.

Your liver can also move said by-products into the bloodstream for further detoxification through the kidneys. Think of this vital organ like your metabolic Buddha. These organs that resemble jumbo beans of the same name are responsible for maintaining balance in the bloodstream. They manage the acid-base ratio of your blood, produce red blood cells when we need them, control and regulate our blood pressure, and keep our electrolyte levels in check. Healthy, functioning kidneys are like the epitome of Zen— they ensure that everything essential in your bloodstream flows in perfect *harmony*. All else that hasn't been repackaged, reused, and repurposed by the powerhouse liver? Buddha takes care of all that—the kidneys work in tandem with some other key anatomical players (heart, lungs, brain—*you may have heard of 'em*) and filter what can still be used to balance blood pressure, pH levels, and hydration status, while excreting anything you can't use via urine.

(*Namaste.*)

All foods contain specific nutrients—vitamins and minerals that are required in certain amounts by the body to do all of the impressive things it is capable of doing in a day. If you're *gorging* on fried food, however, your body will use the fat that it needs and continue metabolizing what it doesn't need through your liver, where by-products are used to create bile or go to your kidneys—and keep repeating that process all day, every day. *I mean, it's like the story line of* Groundhog Day *applied to organ functionality!* But if you switch from mozzarella sticks to cold-pressed detox juice? Your GI tract *still* breaks down that food into its simplest molecular components; your liver *still* assesses, repackages, and repurposes those compounds elsewhere; and your kidneys (and all other implicated organs) *still* balance blood concentration. What's supplied in excess of what you need, no matter the source of those nutrients, will ultimately flow through your bloodstream until it finds where it's needed—and if it's not needed anywhere right now, excess macronutrients ultimately post up in the "storage" system of your body: your fat cells.

Allow me to raise one small but mighty point about jump starts, detoxes, cleanses, and drinking liquids for the purpose of helping your vital organs do what they *already do*: If any of these things worked, wouldn't they be working by now?! Wouldn't 67 percent of people be underweight instead of overweight or obese?

Just a thought; we can all sip on that.

How to Tell If It's Too Good to Be True

So how can you figure out whom to trust when it comes to what's best for your own health and weight? Allow me to don my white cape—I mean *coat*—for a second. This is what dietitians are trained to do: We're trained both in human skills (counseling, motivational interviewing) and in science (biochemistry, organic chemistry, research analytics) to help people find what works for them based on the information we know to be true.

In order to provide evidence-backed nutritional advice, you need the kind of education and training required to be a registered dietitian (RD). Dietitians-in-training attend an accredited university's didactic program in dietetics, which includes learning in the areas of chemistry, biochemistry, food service management, and medical nutrition therapy before they're eligible to apply for a one-year dietetic internship in a hospital that also includes some community- and research-focused work. At the culmination of those—give or take—four years, you still need to pass an exam to become an RD. And if you want to actually *practice*, you'll need a master's or doctoral degree.

Though anyone can call themselves a nutritionist—yes, anyone—your cabdriver, your boss at the firm, or your siblings, without the proper credentials, they are not legally permitted to use the title "registered dietitian." (*Registered dietitians are also nutritionists, though.*)

While there are plenty of people with plenty of fancy certifications and credentials that dispel some pretty inflammatory, contentious, or just generally ill-advised health "advice," it's my job as an RD to help you make healthier choices that work for *you*, using science as the foundation for all recommendations, but with tips on how to actually use them and modify them for your own personal everyday life.

Here's What's Sick About Wellness: It's Just Code for "Diet"

Real talk: I am a health professional, and I'm also of the belief that "wellness" is making us sick, draining our financial resources, and causing an inordinate amount of dissatisfaction and unhappiness. In my opinion, wellness is for today's target consumer (millennials) what high fashion was for the target consumer of the late 1980s and 1990s (everyone). Status is implied if you can afford to buy coconut water laced with algae ($16 for 16 ounces) and if you're able to bend with grace into a "mermaid" (a sit-up, but more torturous) on a Pilates reformer ($41 per fifty-minute class).

In my opinion, all of these hot-spinning, underwater-yoga-ing, charcoal-mainlining fads stand on the shoulders of a history already riddled with diet-culture-induced fear, shame, and self-loathing. "Calorie counting" and "dieting" were the first descriptive terms for efforts to control the types of food to choose and the quantity of food eaten with the goal of losing weight or improving health. When we "failed" (because of a lack of sufficiently *satisfying* information about how and what to eat), we decided *This is too hard! This isn't possible for me!* We never learned enough to understand and implement practices that would make it easier—and continually searched for the next quick fix and magical solution that would just make us feel better about ourselves.

If we really believed we had the agency to take action to lose weight and feel great about our bodies, would we feel like we *had* to love fancy workouts; cold-pressed juice; silent meditation retreats (*It's too HOT to meditate in this desert!*); paleo-"raw"-nola; or gluten-free, dairy-free baked goods otherwise known as *rocks*? I'm not talking about those new workout classes that genuinely bring you joy, or a new food that you *actually really love to cook and eat*; I'm talking about the trendy stuff that you feel like you're *supposed* to be doing because everybody else is getting such *LIFE-CHANGING* results from it. It's these things that cause you to conflate feelings of self-ineptitude with virtuosity, but without empowering yourself to succeed in the first place. Yep—the truth is best served cold.

My distaste for wellness comes from its adjacency to toxic diet behaviors; how competitiveness in a wellness culture can translate into disordered eating habits, weight-cycling, and restriction; and the continued propagation of a myth that in order to be healthy, *you have to be something you're not right now*. That's a shame-trigger. *And it's really not my cup of tea.*

So how do we avoid all that?

Detox Your Mind-Set (Stat!)
Navigating the Information Jungle

6 Questions for Recognizing That You're in the Information Jungle

1. Do I feel overwhelmed or inert when I read/watch/listen to/implement or even *think* about implementing this info?
2. Where is this info coming from? Is it coming from a credible source?
3. Is there consensus around what's being said (e.g., is it coming from a credible source that also supports some preexisting philosophies as well as scientific biologic plausibility, and have enough people been involved in coming to this conclusion to make it worthwhile)?
4. Is this information asking me to eliminate anything?
5. Is there a "jump start," a "detox," or a period of elimination, restriction, or extreme behavior associated with applying this info to my own life?
6. Is there a way that I can try out a small part of this information in my everyday life without completely uprooting my daily routines?

Life in the digital age means that we are constantly maneuvering through questionable advice, skewed results, and a veritable information jungle that can be incredibly difficult to make sense of. It's a jungle out there, and I volunteer to be your guide.

The first obstacle that you might encounter in the info jungle is the state of being overwhelmed. The cause is exposure to a flood of "knowledge," be it evidence-backed or completely baseless/a veritable pile of bs. There are simply too many "flat belly foods," "elimination diets," "diet delivery kits," and claims of "everyday ingredients that are *killing you!*" to keep up with in any reasonable way! In fact, if you really spend much time at all going down the rabbit hole of the internet scavenging for detox diets, you're bound to come away bleary-eyed, exhausted, and confused by all of the obvious contradictions. So if you're in one of these internet holes right now, do yourself a favor: BACK AWAY FROM THE SCREEN.

The other highly contagious epidemic of the information jungle is the perception that achieving better health and losing weight is an extreme sport. Sexy packaging and sneaky marketing make us think that we'll get great results only if we dedicate all of our time, energy, money, and mental health. Achieving better overall health and losing weight seem to require extreme levels of deprivation and restriction that would represent a radical overhaul of the lives we've been living. It's enough to make a person want to just lie down and take an *extreme nap*.

Where Do "Shoulds" Come From?

In the info jungle, two conditions are contagious: Extreme Overwhelm and Extreme Difficulty.

If you've got Extreme Overwhelm, the primary symptom is any degree of anxiety as a result of inundation of conflicting internet facts on how and what to eat, making it impossible to actually eat anything without some level of fear and shame. If you've contracted Extreme Difficulty, the primary symptom is a perception that health improvement of any kind is an Olympic sport that requires Herculean physical (and emotional) effort to put into practice, making it impossible to take any action. I've coined these two conditions because either or both are at the root of "shoulds." These *conditions* reveal themselves through "questions," no matter if you're sitting across from me in an office or emailing me from across the world. Interestingly, they're perceived as questions by those "asking," but they're rarely a question at all! Rather, someone will initiate a conversation with a "should" statement:

- "I know I *should* have a smoothie for breakfast, but I just really don't have the time to make them."
- "I *should* NOT eat sugar, but if it's organic/gluten-free/vegan…"
- "I *should* get an exercise bike, but I just can't afford it right now."
- "I *should* have ordered a salad with dressing on the side instead of a sandwich, but the sandwiches were 50 percent off…"

When you think and say the word *should* as it relates to your diet, you're buying into the notion that *something is wrong with you or something is beyond your control.* (*And, HEY! YOU!! I don't blame you! You're in the info jungle, and it's wild out there!*) By continuously making statements like this, you're telling yourself a version of the same thing: "I must be a *lesser* human being if I can't make this one change that might help to fix my whole life and make me *thin*!"

Unfortunately, what happens in most of these scenarios when we're overwhelmed or feeling particularly vulnerable is shame-inducing all-or-nothing thinking that makes us question our own beliefs and self-worth because of our food choices. The thing about *shoulds* is that the more we tell ourselves what we *should* do, the less likely it becomes that we'll actually do it. *Should* statements create distance between healthful behaviors and what we actually do. They leave us feeling distraught over our perceived ineptitude: We have the answer to our problem; we just lack the ability to follow through. We have all the information we need, but implementing it feels completely intangible and out of reach. *OF COURSE THAT'S DISPIRITING*! So where do we land? Square one, of course. A place of self-loathing, doubt, and repeating the same toxic diet mantra: *I know I should, but...*

The more we keep telling ourselves what we *should* do, followed by what we *can't* do without any reasonable intervention or change, the more we're actually proving ourselves *right*.

Cognitive Distortions, aka "Toxic Diet Thoughts"

Another residual side effect of info jungle–induced Extreme Overwhelm and Extreme Difficulty (besides sadness and a whole lot of time we'll never get back) is something I call "toxic diet thoughts," or TDTs. In my counseling experience, there are two main types of TDTs: ones that elicit self-blame and ones that elicit blame-shifting. Regardless, they're both primed to majorly mess us up—because (a) neither type of thought is true, but both work as mantras that prevent you from taking real action!; and (b) neither of these TDTs *is productive* in helping you make better food choices! (*Which is what you were really trying to do in the first place... right?!*)

I call these thoughts *toxic* because they stem from consistent misinformation and debilitating *confusion*, and they have no place in improving your current state of health and well-being. They're actively holding you captive to your own thoughts, feeling stuck or blaming others, and tricking you into thinking that you don't have the capacity to take control of your own life. In fact, they're making you inert. But what turns them from toxic to *lethal* is when you're saying them inside your head (and even out loud!) so frequently and nonchalantly that you don't ever question their *toxicity level*.

Let's take a minute to familiarize ourselves with and analyze some of these useless statements so we can appropriately *detox from this hellhole of a cognitively distorted dystopia and start living our lives*. Deal?

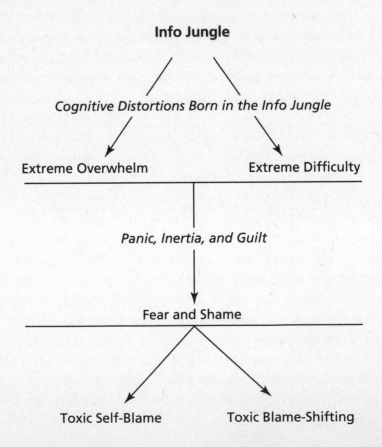

Info Jungle

Cognitive Distortions Born in the Info Jungle

Extreme Overwhelm   Extreme Difficulty

Panic, Inertia, and Guilt

Fear and Shame

Toxic Self-Blame   Toxic Blame-Shifting

Toxic Diet Thoughts from a Perceived Lack of Emotional or Physical Capabilities—→ Cognitive Distortion about Your Own Abilities to Make a Positive Change in Your Health

- *It's too damn hard.*
- *It's too damn confusing.*
- *Something must be wrong with me.*
- *Something must be wrong with the rest of the world; there's nothing wrong with me.*

Self-blame TDTs turn the focus inward, as if you were in a brutal, gloves-off fight with yourself in a mirror. You perceive yourself as the "problem." Most often, self-blame TDTs are a result of being exposed to diet tips, tricks, hacks, and quacks who all seem to be telling you that *you* need more willpower, time, money, and emotional and physical ability to become the person you want to be. Self-blame thoughts tend to start with the phrase "I *can't*":

- "I *can't* eat healthily because doing so requires more time and/or money and/or energy than I have to give right now."
- "I *can't* lose weight because of my current state of health/family history/level of physical fitness."

Just in case this isn't ringing familiar with you just yet, here are some other examples of self-blame toxic diet thoughts :

- "I always gain it back, so what's the point?"
- "I have no willpower."
- "I have no time to do all of the things I'd need to do to lose weight."
- "I don't have the energy to take this on right now."
- "I just can't cut out...(carbs/sugar/fat/gluten/salt/dairy, etc.)."
- "I'm not genetically meant to be thin."

- "I can't give up my entire social life to lose a few pounds."
- "I'm too fat to work out right now."
- "I have no control over my meals."

On the other side of the coin is self-blame's cousin, blame-*shifting*. These TDTs come more from a perception of the outside world as the "problem" and leave you victim to myths that inhibit you from taking real action (and continuously taking action!) by convincing you that something is inherently wrong with the world—leaving you to feel totally helpless (and without agency to *do anything* about it!). These stories find a happy home in the minds of chronic blame-shifters, because they're thoughts that thrive on the fact that it's easier to pass the buck on problems than it is to take ownership of them. When you blame-shift, you give power to things that may not be deserving of such great responsibility, but regardless, they're often things you can't change ("the food industry!") or things you perceive to be *unchangeable* right now ("My kids hate vegetables!"). They all have the same result, though: They make you feel that there's something you *should* be doing, but other people/circumstances/scenarios are the problem—*they're* at fault for getting in the way of your goals. Following are a few examples of blame-shifting TDTs.

Toxic Diet Thoughts from Perceived Lack of Agency or Control→ Cognitive Distortion about the Role of Outside Factors in Impeding Your Progress

- "I'm just totally addicted to sugar!"
- "I should try that new diet, but I'm pretty sure I'm allergic to/intolerant of/my kids won't eat…"
- "Everything I like is toxic."
- "My entire career/office/work schedule/makes it impossible to eat well because…"
- "Drinking and eating are a part of my job."
- "My gym/trainer/workout class is canceled/too far away/too early/too late."

Toxic diet thoughts make you think that you need drastic measures to jump-start yourself to become a completely different person in order to make the changes you want to see. They lead you to feel that everybody on TV and in ads and online is better at this stuff than you are—because there's something wrong with *you*.

First of all, let me say this loud and clear: *THERE IS NOTHING WRONG WITH YOU!*

When you get caught in the info jungle, it's dizzying to know where to start in the fight to get out. (*Trust—we're about to cover most of these, so you'll navigate that info jungle like a champ once we really get under way!!*) Most people either act on misinformation/confusion or don't act at all. It's really complicated and confusing to figure out what is going to make sense for your personal needs. In order to make a *lasting* change, you've got to have the right information, build a healthy amount of confidence connected to *using* said information, and then form a strategy for applying and implementing it in your everyday life. When you carry on sans strategy (or sans *sustainable* strategy, more accurately), you wind up right back in the info jungle—simply because you couldn't *hack the damn wilderness*. But with the right map (information) and the right equipment (attitude and self-confidence), you can make your way out of the information jungle and onto ~~less vegetative~~ more stable ground.

Combating the Info Jungle: Use a Filter

Think of your brain as your mind-set's own bodyguard—a personalized filtration system that empowers you to feel happier and more in control. Just as your liver and your kidneys filter out toxic substances, so, too, is your brain capable of filtering out what is not productive information when it comes to what to eat versus what not to eat. In general, here are the ways you can train yourself to do just that:

First, now that you're here, well...*stay* here! Let's commit to wiping the slate clean—discarding, or at the very least suspending, all of the information you've already been taught about diets, detoxes, and restriction as tools by which to ultimately experience "freedom" from the things in your life that have kept you from losing weight. (PS, has any of that information *ever* worked for you? I *know*. That's why you're here! It works for absolutely *no* one!) At least for the rest of this book, commit to relearning *how* to eat. This can be your mind-set detox!!

(Look! You're jump-starting! Just by reading half of a chapter! Go, you!)

Second: Use a *modified* version of a legal tool known as the Daubert standard, which is used to determine if certain scientific evidence is admissible in a court of law. In legalese, the factors look like this:

- Whether the theory or technique employed by the expert is generally accepted in the scientific community;
- Whether it has been subjected to peer review and publication;
- Whether it can be and has been tested;
- Whether the known or potential rate of error is acceptable; and
- Whether the research was conducted independent of the particular litigation or dependent on an intention to provide the proposed testimony. (In other words, is the research funded by someone with a special interest? Frankly, it's not a universal truth that you need to care if it was, 100 percent of the time. But occasionally when you look deeper into what transpired, the funding provides illustrative context.)

But for you, it can be boiled down to three quick questions to ask yourself when you hear about a new health study, scroll through a blogger's wellness post, or watch news concerning diet and health on any major national network:

1. Does this information or advice make me feel inadequate or overwhelmed?
2. Does this information or advice make me feel better or worse today?
3. Is this information or advice in line with what I like to do, think about, listen to, and learn from every day in a way that feels generally *positive* to me?

If your answers indicate that the information or advice you're considering makes you feel inadequate or overwhelmed, makes you feel worse, or does not feel positive for you, it is not for you. Period. Your modified Daubert standard is a hard-ass, and pseudoscientific information isn't admissible in your personal court of law, aka your *head*.

Three Rules for Adopting New Behavioral Change as It Relates to Your Diet

1. **Know the difference between what "works" and what *works for you*.** Making the change should be challenging enough to get you out of your current routine (and maybe feel slightly *disruptive*)—but not extremely difficult, seemingly impossible, or something that will require you to make major changes to your current activities of daily living.

2. **The only thing you should permanently restrict is *restriction*.** You've probably heard this one a gazillion times, but in this case, we're taking a holistic approach to improvement and taking a definitive stance against restriction. Yes, there will be things you might have to give up *in a given day* to make room for other things *you want more*. And yes, if you find (in chapter 7) that eating Twizzlers at the movies works for you but enjoying Twizzlers in front of your TV at home takes you down a candy rabbit hole, you might try *restricting* that strawberry sugar heaven to a *certain place and time*. But that doesn't mean eliminating an entire food group from your life.

3. **Practice makes confidence. Confidence makes habits, and habits are the building blocks of better health and weight loss.** The more you practice, the more confident you'll be. It's that simple. But in this case, we're not practicing anything fancy—no boot camp (unless you're into that!); no mind games; no thirty-day challenges. You're going to practice *regularly eating solid food*.

Build Confidence with Language: Editing Your Inner Monologue

It's a pet peeve of mine to hear consistent diet-culture language that talks about what you can't eat, do, think, or say rather than what you actually *can* do. Replacing buzzwords with more effective terminology is the perfect place to start building confidence through practice. For our purposes, it's the practice of replacing lesser, more confusing or debilitating or inertia-inducing words with ones that summon a little extra positivity, or flip the script on what's going on inside that info-stuffed head of yours!

Instead of moderation—→ *more*: When it comes to vegetables and fruit? Bottom line is that more is *more* (aka better). Eat more of these foods, and no matter what else you're doing, you're going to lose weight, and you're going to get sick less frequently. Keep this up over time, and you'll also reduce your risk of chronic diseases—not just the common cold.

Instead of elimination—→ *whole*: *Whole* describes the best form in which to eat fiber-filled fruit and veggies. Instead of elimination, think about choosing whole foods more often—fruit instead of fruit juice; vegetables instead of veggie chips; whole-grain bread instead of white bread; a whole baked sweet potato instead of sweet-potato fries. Eating more food in its natural state helps you replace *less nutritious* foods with better ones. This does *not* mean completely eliminating those "less than whole" foods I mentioned, but rather choosing whole foods—and getting creative with how you prepare them—more often.

Instead of "bad food"—→ *treat*: Let's start with the facts. "Bad food" is not a thing. Your liver knows that. Your kidneys know that. The only one who doesn't know that yet is your brain (it's a little slow. *Kidding!*). A "treat" is whatever you personally consider indulgent, which can change from day to day, and it's up to you—not your friends, family members, or coworkers—to assign value to foods you absolutely love but you know would make you feel not so great physically or mentally if you were to eat your weight in them all day, every day.

Instead of "good food"—→ *breakfast, lunch, dinner, snacks*: "Good food" is *also not a thing*, so let's clarify that when we say "good food," we really just mean food that is very much a part of our everyday lives. When we attribute value to food, we're giving it too much power. Remember—food makes up your meals and snacks, which delineate your day and make up other great qualities of your life, depending on whom you're sharing it with. The bottom line: You're the boss of the food you eat. It's not the boss of you. Don't give it so much power by giving a value or a merit award for how many calories, carbs, or grams of sugar it has.

Instead of cheat—→ *eat*: Making mostly value-free food choices means there's no such thing as "cheating." It's not a test you have to ace—*this is your*

LIFE! You eat mostly things you love that you feel work well for you; you indulge in other things you love that make you happy and that taste *good to you*. You're not eliminating anything—except for certain language, like this ugly phrase. No one is grading you at the end of this book, so stop grading (or *degrading*!) yourself for carrying out the biological need of eating food! Real, lasting weight loss is a result of the way that you eat *most of the time*, and it certainly can't be "derailed" by one meal, one day, or one week of eating in a way that's not your personal best. Remember *that*!

Instead of calories⟶ energy: This isn't just a language change; it's a scientific fact: Calories are actually kilocalories, and they're units of energy. The thing to think about *most* here is that because calories are units of energy, they're also what gives you power to do the other things in life you love to do. When you think about how much energy you're getting from a certain food—how it's fueling you to do what's next on your to-do list, or how it provides what you need to do *other things you want to do* (read, walk, go to an exercise class, go out with friends, etc.), you will have a better internal scale of the amount of energy you need to enjoy those activities.

Instead of "I should" and "I can't"⟶"I choose to": Do you live in Maine and wake up in the morning saying, "I'm going to go to Nepal and climb Mount Everest this morning!"? No. Because you *can't actually get to Nepal that quickly*! For the record, that's an example of an instance in which I'm allowing you to use the word *can't*—if it's humanly impossible to do, it's not realistic for you right now (but it might be—if you move to Nepal next year!). *Shoulds*, by contrast, are ascribed notions of what your toxic diet head tells you that you *should do at a certain point in time*, fueled by the notions of others who might be more clueless or misinformed than you! So *shoulds* will have to go (almost) entirely. Instead of saying "I should," say "I choose to." You'll choose to do what's best for you and what aligns with your beliefs. When it doesn't? Well, it's not right for you and it's getting the boot. *Now.*

We're letting in *only the information that serves us*, and we're using only the language that serves our inner monologue! And we're practicing doing just that over and over again—right here, with this book! And we're going to keep on doing it.

It's going to be *so much fun!*

Implement a Strategy: Do Less

If you've ever seen the 2008 movie *Forgetting Sarah Marshall*, you're familiar with this scene. (*PS, if you somehow missed the cultural revelation that is this movie, you may need to put this book down and watch this immediately. Don't worry, I'll wait!*)

Reeling from a traumatic breakup, the main character, Peter, played by Jason Segel, takes a surfing lesson on a beach in Hawaii, where he practices standing up on a surfboard with Paul Rudd's character, Chuck, an ultra-laid-back surfing instructor who goes by "Kunu." Peter attempts to get up on the surfboard by fumbling around clumsily, trying to figure out exactly where to place his long limbs to stand up *just right*, but he winds up stumbling over his own feet, lacking any stability or confidence (all while still on the sand—not even in the ocean). Kunu, albeit stoned to infinity, watches Peter and provides feedback: "You're doing too much," he says. "Do less."

Through my work with patients, clients, and readers, the number one greatest overarching mistake I see is this: *Everyone is trying to force changes into their diets by doing too much all at once and without any real stability!* And guess what happens? We *can* lose weight—in the way Peter *can* flail and stumble to his feet on the surfboard while thinking about every muscle movement and limb placement (which continuously backfires!). But as Kunu so, er, *aptly* recognizes: If even the smallest wave were to hit Peter while he's out there stumbling around on that surfboard trying to find his footing, he'd collapse. And the same applies to our efforts to lose weight.

Yes, there are *tons* of scientific evidence supporting *why* different diets *can* work. But my experience has taught me that most of us are just like Peter on the surfboard: We are completely in our own heads about how to lose weight and we don't have a solid foundation to keep us strong and grounded in the face of a wave (for our purposes, that's literally any and every life event, big or small, on any given day of the week). We're all Peter, belly-flopped on a Hawaiian surfboard (*our emotional rock bottom, am I right?!*), overwhelmed by *feelings* of failure (because of the countless diets we've been on to lose weight, only to eventually gain it all right back), and trying to get up again (go on another diet to lose weight)—not recognizing the real problem: We've heard, read, and watched *too much already*; we're doing too much *right now*, and we're doing it without a shred of strategy! So color me Kunu:

DO LESS! Your first strategic step is to stop counting calories and trying to make too many changes all at once.

We'll start the next chapter with more actionable strategies to go with your new "do less" mind-set. But if any strategy feels like too much, too soon (I don't think it will, but just to be sure we're *crystal* on this one): *Don't do it*! Try modifying or scaling back on a strategy to make it feel more like 80 percent attainable and 20 percent aspirational to you. Once you've done *that* for a week? You'll add another one. And so on, and so on...

Sounds simple, right? It is. You'll be *doing less* than you were before you picked up this book! You're going to learn to think and say positive things about food, and then you're going to *actually* eat it—*consistently*!

(I'm having so much fun already!)

2

I Have No Willpower

In this chapter, you'll learn...

- why willpower won't work;
- how to replace feelings of paralysis with real, tangible action;
- how to make a satisfying breakfast (at home or on the go); and
- how to practice accountability to keep yourself feeling satisfied, not just full.

Your strategy for better health habits starts with eating regular meals and snacks—because (a) every time you eat, you have another chance to *practice* making better choices and becoming more confident in your own abilities to change your state of health, and (b) food is *delicious*! Plus, it keeps you alive, which is *key* if we're going to get some sh*t done around here.

We've all heard the same old tropes:

Eat when you're hungry; stop when you're full! Eat six small meals per day! Eat, but only until 4 p.m.! Don't eat, just drink liquids! Try not to eat until around 4 p.m., when you may have a cube of cheese if you feel like you might pass out! (Emily Blunt in *The Devil Wears Prada*, anyone?!)

In the tangled web of the info jungle, there's a whole lot of messaging telling us to *stop eating*. Don't-eat-isms that appear in signals we've received throughout our lives—from family, friends, news articles, reporters, celebrities, social media, and even good old-fashioned science—have been telling us somewhat covertly (*and in the case of many family members, very overtly*) that we should all be flipping on some magical little switch inside ourselves to activate *willpower*, the antidote to *enjoying food* that all of us can simply access—if only we could *just stay strong enough*!

If the aforementioned words of advice were really working for you, would you feel the way you're feeling right now? Wouldn't you have thought at some point over the years, *Wow! Portion control is mind-blowing!!! What a novel concept! I'm going to eat less and it's going to make me lose weight, and everything will be amazing!*

There's quite a lot of contradictory scientific literature out there (e.g., six small meals versus intermittent fasting), but for the most part, science provides the obvious conclusions: When you eat matters exponentially *less* than how much you eat in a day (how many total units of energy—calories—you take in versus expend in a twenty-four-hour period). Whether or not meal frequency plays a role in your body's own metabolic rate is highly individualized. And other lifestyle-related factors—for example, you eat ice cream during the 5 p.m. news every day, or you exercise during the 5 p.m. news every day—play a role in determining how you use versus store energy.

Willpower simply provides you with a Band-Aid coping mechanism that sets you up to nearly *hate yourself* when you mess up in the slightest, because "messing up" in the context of having willpower feels a lot like we're telling ourselves how lazy and inept we are. It's *so mean! You're not strong enough to skip bread? WHAT IS WRONG WITH YOU?!* Willpower can get you through *certain* scenarios, such as when you're grocery shopping and resist loading up your cart when you walk by the bakery aisle because you know you're reaching for that stuff only because it's lunchtime and you're hungry. But what about when you're trying *so hard not to eat cake* that you avoid it the first time around because of *willpower*, but then you wake up the next day and still all you can think about is that *f*cking cake*, which you're trying not to eat *any of ever again*, so maybe having whipped cream on your morning latte will help you stop thinking about cake, but *OMG is it seriously Linda's BIRTHDAY in the office?!* So then you eat cake, and *everything else* on the birthday treat table you "shouldn't eat."

This makes you feel like you "have no willpower" and that you have to restrict yourself *even more*, when, really, willpower got you into that situation to begin with.

The problem with trying to use willpower to change the way you eat is that it teaches you to suffer through situations that you can actually prevent from happening in the first place simply by eating real food, and doing so regularly. The idea of using only willpower to stop you from eating precludes you from actually learning about yourself and understanding why you want something in a given moment. Ultimately, it's a quick fix because it can (occasionally) work in the present, but it provides zero information that you can use to inform your future.

Willpower: A Means to a Future Self?

Willpower plays on the misguided belief that if you restrict or deny yourself certain foods, you will achieve some sort of destiny where you're suddenly thin, beautiful, healthy, and, most importantly—happy. But this doesn't actually work! Achieving goals that you've set for yourself is great—but when the sole focus is restriction for the sake of weight loss, you lose sight of the reasons why you'd like to lose weight in the first place—health, self-assurance and self-gratitude (feelings that can develop when you feel your best!), and building confidence that creates a sustainable foundation for your present self and your future self.

The more we focus on restraint as a means to achieve said goals, the less we prioritize our bodies and our physical and mental states of health, right? If we're constantly depriving ourselves in order to get to the next *thing*, we're not teaching ourselves how to actually live as the version of ourselves we want to be. We're not creating a strategic plan for how losing weight and being healthier will look, feel, and actually help us.

If Not Willpower, Then What?

Energy balance is the idea that the energy from the food you consume in a day is equal to the energy your body needs to operate over the course of a twenty-four-hour period. In order to achieve weight loss, you have to actually use up more energy, or calories, than you've taken in—*negative energy balance*—a concept traditional diets feed off by relying on principles of calorie restriction and limitation. All diets, even when they're dressed up in cute little costumes like paleo and keto and cabbage soup, are relying on the same idea: calories in, calories out. Eat more than you burn, and you'll gain weight. Eat less than you burn, and you'll lose weight. The programs apply different strategies to get you to eat less and take in fewer calories by focusing on how much you're eating of certain foods.

The problem here is that these programs don't consider the many other factors that impact a person's ability to sustain the practice of eating fewer calories. Namely, *satiety*.

There's a fair amount of data to suggest that, in terms of our own personal motivation and resolve, we diminish our willpower reserve over the course of a day. But in the context of health and weight loss, the idea that willpower decreases over the course of the day may be a factor, but it's only a piece of the puzzle. The definition of it shows us why: We need *food* in order to live. If we don't eat food consistently, in the right combination of nutrients that satisfy us, and stay aware and on top of other biological factors that play a role in appetite regulation, guess what happens? *You want all of the things you were restricting! You want them more than EVER! And it's damn near impossible to resist because you're trying to exercise an emotional muscle on an empty stomach! (And really, there's basically nothing you should do on an empty stomach. Except for maybe swimming, according to your grandma. Or getting a colonoscopy.)*

*Biological Sh*t Starters*

Let's start by going back to biology basics: What we *do* know, based on decades of research, is that three factors play significant roles in people's appetites, how much or how often we feel like eating, and how much we'll actually burn on a day-to-day basis, aka energy balance (calories in, calories out):

1. Sleep
2. Physical activity
3. Hydration status

Beyond the fact that you're about to get yourself a strategy and a framework for healthier eating, these three factors are some of the most understated yet prominent influences on how much you eat and what you burn every day. So even if you ignore all of the other strategies on these pages, bringing awareness to these three aspects of your own personal biology provides you with some context for why negative energy balance (burning more than you consume) can feel hard sometimes. (*It's not your "lack of willpower"! It's human biology! Isn't that so reassuring?!*)

ENERGY BALANCE 101

Resting Energy Expenditure (REE)

- REE accounts for 60–75 percent of twenty-four-hour energy expenditure.
- REE is involuntary energy expended by the body at rest to keep vital organ systems functioning and basically keep you alive.
- REE is manipulated by your *level* of physical fitness (aka how strong you are) but not determined by the type of exercise you do in a day; it is based mostly on genetics.

Thermic Effect of Food (TEF)

- TEF accounts for 10–15 percent of twenty-four-hour energy expenditure.
- TEF is the energy used by your body to digest, absorb, and metabolize what you eat, a factor that's only minimally affected by physical activity.
- TEF energy expenditure is minimally affected by physical activity.

Physical-Activity-Related Energy Expenditure

- Physical activity accounts for 20–35 percent of twenty-four-hour energy expenditure.
- Physical-activity-related energy is expended in voluntary body movements in daily activities, sports, play, and some nonvoluntary behaviors (e.g., fidgeting, muscle contractions).

- Physical-activity-related energy is what you expend in voluntary movement (exercise, taking Fido for a walk, socializing, activities of daily living, and so on) and some nonvoluntary ones (like fidgeting and muscle contractions).

Sleep

The less sleep you get, the hungrier you're likely to feel. In fact, sleeping less than seven hours per night is linked to increased appetite; decreased energy expenditure (how many calories you burn in a day); altered glucose metabolism (blood sugar abnormalities); risk of weight gain over time; and other long-term health complications, so it's important for us to be mindful of our sleep needs.

Lack of good, quality sleep affects your appetite-regulating hormones, leptin and ghrelin, which are responsible for telling you when you're full (the former goes *down*) versus hungry (the latter goes *up*), depending on how rested you are. Plus, lack of sleep also has been linked to increased insulin production, decreased insulin sensitivity, and a rise in blood sugar (aka the way your body responds to digestion and absorption of food you eat)—all of which, when looked at across population studies, have been linked to type 2 diabetes, cardiovascular disease, and overall mortality.

(Sounds scary, right? But don't worry—there's an upside.)

Sleep is a necessity, and making it a priority is a goal for many—especially those who have read Arianna Huffington's brilliant book *The Sleep Revolution*. But our relationship with sleep, similar to dietary preferences and feelings about food, also varies greatly depending on current phase of life (a shout-out to new parents everywhere!) and plenty of other factors that we often feel we aren't able to directly control (again, new parents, caretakers, and *roommates* everywhere—*I hear you!*). And as someone who doesn't even remember what it's like to get seven hours of sleep per night on a regular basis (I'm *working on it!*), I can 100 percent empathize with all of you four-hour-a-nighters who think that getting seven hours is completely impossible for you.

For the purposes of this book, I'm not going to focus all that much on changing your sleep patterns—we are here to talk about changing your eating habits after all! But the key takeaways from research are important to keep in mind as we move through these strategies for forming better habits. If you're not aware of the fact that there are *other reasons* why you might be feeling like it's tough to get a handle on what you eat in a day, then it's easy to just put the blame on your lack of impulse control.

My point is that whether or not you want to change your sleep habits is up to you—but it's my job to let you know that:

- your nightly z's aren't stagnant—absolutely everyone has sleep disruptions at one time or another;
- if you're feeling more tired and hungry than usual, you might just consider a nap (if that's an option); and
- if you know you haven't gotten enough sleep, you're more likely to feel hungry and it's less likely that the ol' "willpower" Band-Aid will work as it normally would when you're more rested; therefore, it's worth considering how to prepare in advance so you feel empowered—not powerless.

#protip

Being sleep-deprived is a primer for feeling powerless against cookies, cake, and whatever else you've convinced yourself requires *more willpower* to resist. It's not about muscling through it; it's literally about sleeping *more*, on a more consistent basis—whatever that means for *you*—which is right in line with your whole "do less" mentality.

I don't give you this information to make you feel bad or to add another thing to your list of "Things I'm Doing Wrong." Knowledge is power, and it's important to understand the real reasons your body is craving what it's craving so you can be more aware of your feelings-turned-into-actions surrounding your own eating habits.

PREPPING FOR "FATIGUE-EATING"

The first step in staying on top of fatigue-eating is to *know* and *be aware* that you're fatigue-eating.

We'll get into specifics of how to stay prepped for other food scenarios in your daily life, but for now, snacks that specifically help to battle fatigue-eating have three components:

1. They're volume-based (meaning you can eat a lot at a lower "calorie-cost").
2. They're crunchy (we tend to crave crunchy foods more when we're tired and exhausted).
3. They have a comfort-food quality (something you might've wanted to eat as a kid when you were home sick or needed a little extra TLC).

Examples of snacks to pack for the Battle of the Nosh: a bag of flavored popcorn (about 4 cups); pea crisps (such as Harmless Harvest or World of Peas); frozen grapes or berries; cherry tomatoes; apples (whole or in slices); bean-based chips; dried cheese crisps; freeze-dried fruit; pre-sliced veggies; whole-grain cereal (like Cheerios).

Physical Activity

A 2016 article in *Obesity Reviews* looked at data on weight and exercise and concluded something we've all considered quite *obvious* for centuries: Physical activity and diet are like birds of a feather. There's tremendous value placed on exercise these days, which has probably contributed to the rise in popular, boutique fitness studios and a whole new metric in the fashion industry otherwise known as *athleisure*. Across all research, regular exercise—defined as physical exertion above and beyond your normal state of movement—of about four hours per week is linked to weight maintenance. Regular exercisers, in conjunction with other dietary factors, often lose weight *not* because of how many calories they burn in a workout (in fact, it's not all that much in the context of your day, though it depends on the type, duration, and intensity) but because of how much their appetite is affected by their activity level, and above all else: how regular exercise helps you build momentum on any goal—especially health-related ones. The secret ingredient in this health and weight-loss recipe? *Consistency.*

Your appetite hormones are directly affected by exercise type and intensity—ghrelin, your "hunger hormone," is *suppressed* right after you do something strenuous, and leptin, your "satiety hormone" (along with peptide YY, glucagon-like peptide 1, and pancreatic polypeptide—don't worry, there's no quiz at the end of this) is increased. How long that appetite suppression lasts depends on the intensity and duration of your workout. While straight cardio (aerobic activity—like running or cycling) tends to suppress ghrelin and peptide YY, anaerobic exercise (like weight lifting or barre) mostly suppresses ghrelin (not so much the peptide YY). Regardless, the suppression seems to take effect after sixty to ninety minutes of said exercise (the greater the intensity, the greater the appetite suppression!). So if you're taking a fifteen-minute casual stroll on the treadmill, you might not experience any *I can't possibly eat this bagel!* feelings.

We'll touch on exercise a little bit more later on, but for now, the bottom line: You may feel less of a need to graze if you're exercising regularly; you may also feel *more* of a propensity to graze if you exercise regularly—particularly if you're doing a lot of aerobic exercise (aka cardio). Keep this in mind as you become more aware of your personal response to different types of physical activity or eating schedules, and how that response relates to what you eat every day. If an early morning long run (one mile for some, twenty miles for others) makes you absolutely ravenous and ready to eat the contents of your fridge, that's not a lack of willpower—that's your body responding to your appetite hormones postexercise. Similarly, you may not feel like eating at all after some Barry's Bootcamp sprints, but twelve hours later you're scavenging for postdinner protein bars in the depths of your kitchen cabinets.

There's a lot of confusion in regard to exercise and how it affects both weight loss and how much energy you burn—and a huge reason for that is we fail to look at the big picture of what "regular exercise" actually means: It's just another way of saying, "Be regular and consistent with whatever you choose to do!" Doing physically active things you enjoy regularly to the point where you don't want to sleep through them means you are consistently committing to making an exercise-related lifestyle change—so there's no reason to "sweat it" if you work out super hard one day and take the next day off. The more consistent you are over time, the more predictable your appetite becomes—which makes it easier to plan ahead.

Hydration

Many (if not *all*) of my clients confuse thirst with hunger. Interestingly, staying hydrated seems to be one of those (very rare) *shoulds* that are actually worthwhile: Proper hydration is key not only to making sure we stay alert and energized, but also to keeping everything functioning in our bodies. Most of us need to drink between eight and ten cups (as a general rule of thumb) of water per day—and much more when we factor in heat, sweat (even if you don't exercise—sleep sweats count, too!), medications, and humidity shifts. The guideline is loosely based on an equation that determines milliliter per calorie consumed per day, but even if you're eating much more or far less daily, it's a good barometer to think of 2,000 milliliters or 2 liters (about 8 cups) as a middle-ground benchmark.

#protip

Our thirst-alert mechanism declines as we grow older (another *lovely* side effect of aging!), so it's ideal to make drinking water regularly a priority *now*.

Dehydration can produce a number of different side effects, from feeling a little lethargic to plummeting blood pressure. While everyone's sweat rate is different, it's safe to assume that for every forty-five to sixty minutes of exercise you do, you'll need to drink a *minimum* of 40 ounces of H_2O—a number that will probably seem to be staggeringly *high* to some of you.

How to Hydrate 101

Wake Up and Drink

If you're sleeping you're (presumably) *not* drinking, so it's likely that you're waking up in a state of subclinical dehydration. Start your day with a little refreshment in the form of 16 ounces of water—*right away.* Keeping a 16-ounce container of water on your nightstand or putting out a glass before bed to fill in your kitchen in the morning helps. Any visual cue will help you stay on top of it.

Replenish Losses

If you're walking frequently or are a frequent exerciser, rehydration isn't just about water—it's also crucial to get back those electrolytes, like sodium, potassium, and, in lesser amounts, calcium and magnesium, that are responsible for the fluid-electrolyte balance of your cells (a factor that plays a role in basically all bodily functions and in keeping your body working the way it's supposed to).

Caffeine Counts

Here's a little-known fact: Unsweetened beverages such as coffee and tea "count" toward your daily hydration goal—and can be a tasty upgrade without the *snooze* of plain ol' water. Another benefit: Coffee and tea have more recently been linked to reducing risk of chronic disease thanks to their high antioxidant profile, and caffeine (the USDA Dietary Guidelines recommend 300–400 mg per day—or about 3–4 cups of coffee) may lend a hand in both short- and long-term cognition and sharpening memory.

Sparkling Counts, Too

Good news for LaCroix enthusiasts—sparkling water, seltzer, and club soda will help you hydrate, too! Choose flavored or plain options and drink with abandon. The only time to skip these bubbles is if you feel that they're making you bloated or gassy, or if you're choosing a brand with a higher amount of trace sodium (common in sparkling bevs imported from outside of the United States). Types to limit a bit more: brands with acesulfame-K, stevia, or sucralose. Research supports these sweeteners as being safe as part of a healthful diet, but they can exacerbate the bloat-inducing effects of bubbles.

When in Doubt: Produce

Just one apple, for example, can pack up to ½ cup of H_2O; plus, it's got loads of vitamin C, fiber, and phytonutrients (all key for health). Snack on extra veggies with hummus or salsa, add an extra heap of tomatoes to a salad, and get generous with your serving sizes of berries, citrus, melon, grapes, and whatever fruits you love. Another #protip: Add fruit to regular or sparkling water (frozen fruit works for this, too!). It'll add flavor and deliver an extra hit of fiber.

#protip

Hydration Hacks

These unsweetened caffeinated beverages "count" toward your fluid needs:

Iced cold brew coffee

Iced matcha

Latte with nonfat milk or unsweetened soy milk

Coffee with sugar-free syrup

Hot or iced tea with lemon or lime wedges

Hot or iced black tea, unsweetened or sugar-free (e.g., Diet Snapple)

Tea with nonfat milk or unsweetened soy milk

Caffeinated seltzer (like Hiball and Hint waters)

Bai5, CORE, VitaminWater Zero

Biology + Self-Awareness = No More "White-Knuckling It"

In order to create a strategy that empowers us to have ownership over food choices (and to make decisions that are good for us both physically and mentally!), we need to understand what our patterns actually are. We have to be aware of what kind of scenario makes us want a particular meal or snack, and what we're doing while we're eating it, how we feel before we eat, what we feel while we eat, and how we feel after we've finished. When we do tune in to what *else* is going on in our lives before, during, and after we eat? That's when the magic happens. Knowing ourselves—our patterns within the framework of our everyday lifestyles—we're automatically better served because we can actually *tangibly* practice letting food preferences *inform* choices that make us feel good right now, in a few hours, and in a few years.

That's why it's time to break down a few of the most commonly ignored (and completely detrimental!) biological factors and eating *patterns* that almost always interfere with people's ability to practice making conscious food choices that cultivate confidence—patterns that have less to do with *hunger* and everything to do with your response to your hunger. Becoming self-aware when it comes to food choices—and noticing what you're doing without *judging* yourself for doing it—can help you move on to bigger and better things (like actually choosing to eat dessert instead of grazing leftover Tootsie Rolls from your kids' Halloween stash.

(Doesn't that sound so much better to you?! I know, me too.)

"Willpower" Sh*t Starters

In today's diet culture, *not eating* and *not holding yourself accountable* seem to be the two greatest sh*t starters to achieving weight loss and maintaining it long-term.

Often when we eat because of our feelings or perceive certain desires as food "cravings" (and subsequently shame ourselves for lacking "willpower"), it is *not* actually because we can't resist the temptation of a cookie. It's because we're going into battle with our demons without any armor or weapons to defend ourselves! And trying to win a war with personal demons on an empty stomach is *impossible*! Practicing good habits builds confidence in regularly making satisfying food choices and letting it be okay to "mess up."

In initial sessions with clients, I *always find* that one of these three reasons (or a combination of all three in the same day!) fuels overeating, or tricks people into believing that they have "no willpower," when really it's got absolutely zero to do with *anything*! *These factors are basically sh*t starters of your own that spiral into actually believing this bs story you've been telling yourself for decades!* Let's take a look:

- Not eating enough at breakfast (or no breakfast at all).
- Skipping the meal (or snack) before this one... or the one before that.
- Not being accountable to anything or anyone—including (and *especially*) not being self-accountable.

How do you combat these little sh*t starters? You need some immediate, Right-Now Rules: You can start following them immediately, and they require minimal effort. Think of these three things as being like the thermal undies you'd wear if you were going to climb Mount Everest (if you *can* get to Nepal... and if you're into that sort of thing...): If you have *those* on, your first layer of protection is *set*. Everything will (eventually!) have to be handled while ascending—possible avalanches, the Sherpa's whereabouts, where you're going to poop... but we can figure that out *later*. For now, we have to be as prepared as possible to combat freezing temperatures. Make sense? Good. Let's start suiting up.

Right-Now Rule #1: Eat Regularly

Sounds basic, no? But actually, it's not! How do I know that? Because, dear readers, you told me so! All of you are out there, not eating regularly, skipping lots of meals (and definitely skipping some satisfying snacks!), and diving into take-out tater tots at 4 p.m.! In fact, here are some of the most common reasons you've told me about why you "just can't!" when it comes to eating regularly:

- "I had no time!"
- "It was too early!"
- "It was too close to bedtime."
- "It was too close to lunchtime."
- "It was too close to dinnertime."
- "I didn't know what to eat!"
- "I had nothing with me to eat!"
- "I was about to faint and all I could find was a pack of pretzels."
- "I was in a meeting and I couldn't eat in there/the cafeteria was closed after the meeting ended."
- "I forgot!"
- "I was too stressed/sad to eat!"

Timing, Type, and Tools: The Three T's of Better, Smarter, More Successful Strategizing

The three T's are my go-to strategy for overall guidelines on when to eat, what to eat, and how to make sure you're doing it right in ways that uphold your own personal goals. It's super effective because, first of all, alliteration is fun! And also, it provides a framework for the types of things to think about at every meal, and the nutrients you need to make any eating occasion more satisfying, and it liberates you to plan your own meals and snacks based on your personal calendar. The tools you'll build in to keep the first two *in practice* are simple and can be done anywhere, anytime.

1. **Timing:** Every three to four hours. Regular snacking is the key to sticking with Right-Now Rule #1. In order to actually do this, you have to know your daily calendar and recognize some details about your daily schedule so you can plan ahead for any potential stretches of time that could lead you to skip a meal or a snack. But since timing is now a huge component of how you're going to stop using the will-power crutch to "power through" your day and starve until you can face-plant into happy hour snacks, you have to make eating regularly a priority. How do you do that? Use the alarm clock on your phone. Have a little "ding" go off every four hours (max) to remind you that it's time to snack. This is also a tremendously helpful tool if you

(a) need to pee during a presentation, (b) cannot listen to Bob from accounting talk about pension for another second, or (c) want to check social media because it's been *four f*cking hours*, Bob. Can we wrap this up? Keeping snacks on hand will help you make it through.

2. **Type:** When it comes to your plate, here's how you're going to start designing your meals and thinking about lunch and dinner—no matter where you are in the world and whatever else you're doing, your plate can and will look this way: mostly veggies (at least 50 percent, but vegetables are an unlimited food for you—so fill 'er up!); lean protein, like fish, seafood, poultry, lean cuts of beef, eggs, tofu; some carbs from beans, lentils, chickpeas, peas (those are top preferences), or starchy veggies (tubers and other potatoes, whole grains). There should also be some good hearty fats on your plate, so you can actually stay satisfied throughout the day: avocado; seeds or nuts (about ¼ to ⅓ cup, or a 1-ounce pack, on top of whatever you're eating); cheese (because it makes everything better, and also packs up to 9 g protein per 1-ounce serving).

3. **Tools:** Keep a list in your phone of three go-to places from which you can always grab and go with a nutritious meal that combines all the things listed above under "Type." Use a food-delivery app on your phone to save meal options that can be reordered. This is a brilliant tool to use with the intent of sticking to a healthful eating plan for a given meal during the day rather than scrolling through options and ultimately choosing a huge serving of cheese fries.

Right-Now Rule #2: Build a Better Breakfast (and Eat It Every Day)

Let me know if any of these sentences sound familiar to you:

- "I don't eat breakfast because I drive my kids to school and I would need something I could eat with one hand."
- "I just have coffee with cream for breakfast."
- "I don't have time for breakfast."
- "I grab some fast food on my way to the office."

- "I don't want to eat breakfast because then I've wasted my calories for the day."
- "Once I've prepped my entire family's meals/snacks for the day and gotten everyone out the door, I need a nap, not food!"
- "I just have a smoothie (or green juice) for breakfast."
- "I'm never hungry in the morning."
- "If I eat breakfast, I'm hungrier for lunch, but when I don't, I can go the whole day without eating 'til dinner."
- "I wake up so early it feels ridiculous to eat breakfast when it's dark outside, so I wait 'til I get to the office and by then I'm ravenous."
- "I have no idea what to eat for breakfast."

The other thing that all of my clients who have used all of these phrases have in common? Once they started eating a better, bigger, higher-nutrient-quality breakfast, *literally all of them* lost weight. Yes, really—and I'm pretty certain that's not a coincidence.

Bingeing happens for a whole slew of reasons, but most of us are at our peak level of susceptibility when we're feeling particularly vulnerable to a takedown via *our own thoughts*, and on a (somewhat) empty stomach. You feel crappy, so you start beating yourself up. Next, you start eating for reasons that are seemingly elusive to you and subsequently kick yourself for doing *that*. "I'm the worst!" you say, while hoovering reheated Thanksgiving pie from the freezer. And then you beat yourself up mentally over that, too (shame spirals *suck*!).

Here's the truth: All of this could have been avoided if you'd just had a *sensible breakfast*. Starting off the day with a full, nutrient-dense meal allows you to keep making better choices throughout the day, and also has the unique effect of zapping the "I can't stop eating late at night!" feelings that creep into our brains and lead us right to the kitchen for a stale Tootsie Roll takedown. (*Aren't we learning so much already?!*)

Breakfast 101

There is a large body of epidemiological evidence that consistently supports the idea that consuming breakfast leads to better overall health and a lower body mass index (BMI). While different trials have gotten different results, there *is* one major takeaway from all types of breakfast-related research that we can use to our benefit.

Across the research landscape, there's no evidence that anyone is *gaining weight by eating breakfast*!! What does that mean for you? Even in the *worst-case scenario*, eating breakfast regularly is linked to weight *maintenance*. Why is that? Because most of the evidence suggests that you're likely to burn more calories throughout the day after having a big breakfast, while *skipping* breakfast is linked to burning fewer calories throughout the day—negating any weight-loss benefit of taking in fewer calories to begin with. (*Patterns, people!*)

All things being equal, research *universally* supports one foolproof fact: It is better to have eaten breakfast and *not lost* (weight) than to *never have eaten it at all*!

What the F*ck Do I Even Eat for Breakfast?!

You always need a first meal of the day—but *when* you eat depends on your body, your schedule, and what time you wake up in the morning. Regardless of all of that, breakfast needs to be three things:

1. In your life—every single day (you already knew that!)
2. A combination of fiber and protein (with some fat in there—I'll show you how that works in a sec)
3. Bigger (size *does matter*...at least in breakfast)

Focusing on number 3 for a minute: How do I *know* your breakfast isn't big enough? Well, because I have experience: If you're anything like anyone I've *ever counseled on weight loss*, the odds are really high that if you *are* actually eating this meal, you're not eating enough satisfying stuff *during it*.

#protip

Hard-boiled eggs are great to store anywhere you'll find yourself eating food during the day (aka in a fridge at your office or at home). If you don't want to boil them yourself, you can buy packages of hard-boiled eggs to take on the go (bonus: Many of these are already peeled!!). While there might be a slight markup, they can be well worth the investment. Eating hard-boiled eggs on toast, on the side with fruit, or as part of leftover stir-fry at your morning meal can cut way down on prep time and maximize nutrition density (2 eggs = 16 g of protein!).

A good breakfast should combine protein, stick-to-your-ribs fat, and some fiber-filled carbs; this is your key to feeling satisfied, energized, and *not* ready to eat your stapler by lunch. And since I tend not to focus all that much on calories (so that you're not all kinds of *hung up on counting those*—c'mon, readers, *DO LESS!*), I want you to think of it this way instead: To make any of the breakfast combos suggested below heartier, go up on the veggies and/or the fruit—these are *unlimited* as far as I'm concerned, especially at breakfast. In fact, let's repeat that one: Produce. Is. Unlimited. If you're already a breakfast eater and you *know* that adding more veggies and fruit isn't going to make you feel any more satisfied, then it's pretty likely that you're not getting enough protein at breakfast, so double up (an extra egg, more nuts/nut butter/leftover chicken—you get the picture).

STOP TRYING TO "MAKE" BREAKFAST

Sometimes, it's just not gonna happen. So let's really do less here, shall we? Think about "organizing" breakfast instead of "making" breakfast. Use freezer staples, portable fridge contents, and portable pantry staples (even if perishable—you have minimum two hours before there's any risk of spoilage, which is likely a nonissue for anyone/everyone not living in Los Angeles. *Might be wise to keep a cooler in that Prius, bro!*). Another clutch aspect of mastering breakfast to go: condiments.

- 2 frozen 100 percent whole-grain waffles with 1 tablespoon peanut butter, plus 1 cup berries of choice.
- 2 eggs on a slice of 100 percent whole-grain toast with ½ of an avocado and ½ cup tomatoes; add salt and pepper to taste.

- ½ to 1 cup cooked oatmeal with ½ cup milk of choice, plus 2 to 3 table-spoons mixed nuts (or 1 to 2 tablespoons nut butter of choice), plus 1 piece of fruit.
- ½ to 1 cup Greek yogurt with 1–2 cups berries of choice, plus 2 table-spoons nut butter.
- ½ to 1 roasted (or nuked!) sweet potato with ½ tablespoon nut butter, plus sliced apple/pear/banana.
- Last night's leftover veggies, plus 2 hard-boiled eggs.

Foods you can eat with *one hand* include bananas (and other fruits like apples, peaches, pears, plums); nut butter packs (Justin's, Barney Butter, PB Crave, Wild Friends, and Buff Bake—these are all squeeze packs, so you can vacuum them up while also holding a subway pole); and, of course, bars, which are all 100 percent real food and range in calories from 110 to 250, so they provide an assortment of basic options that you can build upon.

#protip

Make your caffeine count: Ordering an unsweetened latte with low-fat, nonfat, or unsweetened soy milk is an easy way to maximize your mode of caffeination—and make your coffee work overtime for you. A Starbucks Grande (16-ounce cup) contains about 13 grams of protein if you add one of these milks, with minimal saturated fat and no added sugar (as long as you're going unsweetened). Pair this with other items you can buy, like a 1- to 1.5-ounce pack of trail mix (look for versions that have unsweetened fruit as their primary fruit ingredient!) or a piece of fruit (if you're planning on eating more at the office); or add a 200- to 250-calorie bar to the mix to satisfy you through the morning (such as RX Bar, KIND Nuts and Spices, Nature Valley Protein, or Lärabar).

Breakfast in Two Parts

This strategy gives you small bites of (filling) freedom. First, it allows you to complete your Right-Now Rule #1, eating breakfast every day. Second, it lets you eat in *places other* than your dining room or at your kitchen counter. And last, it also maximizes flavor and minimizes time. Behold: This is a sample breakfast meal plan based on one received from a former client who started work at either 6 a.m. or 7 a.m., depending on an alternating schedule (the two-part breakfast is *key* if your day starts in what most of us might consider the middle of the *night*!).

Part 1

Aim for about 100 calories before you get to the office, based on your start time that day:

Take these on the go, and grab your usual nonfat latte:

- Lärabar Minis (I like the peanut butter chocolate chip! But the apple pie is legit, too).
- Breakstone's Cottage Cheese (not a problem for that to sit at room temp for one to two hours…just wouldn't exceed that two-hour mark).
- Chobani or Siggi's yogurt tubes (for real—they come in yummy flavors and they're so easy to pack/won't spoil!).
- Eden Foods 1-ounce package Montmorency dried tart cherries.

Part 2

Try any combo of fiber (whole grains, veggies, fruit) with protein (egg whites, lox, cottage cheese, plain yogurt). Go-tos:

- Bagel with schmear.
- Thomas' 100% Whole Wheat Bagel Thin with a literal schmear (1 to 2 tablespoons) of Philadelphia Whipped Cream Cheese, 3 to 4 ounces of lox (a few slices!), and tomato, onions, cucumber—and whatever

other veg you want on there! And 100 percent whole wheat English muffins are great, too.

- Cinnamon French toast.
- Cinnamon bagel thin (or English muffin) with ½ cup cottage cheese, 1 tablespoon of jelly/honey/apple or pumpkin butter/apple butter with cinnamon.
- Open-faced grilled cheese.
- 1 bagel thin or English muffin topped with ½ cup cottage cheese, sliced tomatoes, peppers; nuke on high for 20 seconds; top with onions, more veggies, et cetera. (I know microwaving sounds absurd with cottage cheese, but it makes it just melty enough to give a little grilled cheese essence.)
- Egg-white omelet with veggies.
- Lots of veggies; scrambled egg whites; turkey; a sprinkle of mozzarella; 1 to 2 slices of whole-grain bread.

Cheesy Toppings

- Use around ⅓ cup if cheese is a big part of whatever you're making and is the only source of protein in the meal (like a homemade veggie bowl/warm salad or veggie soup).
- Use ¼ cup of cheese if it's for adding flavor.
- Use ¼ cup part-skim cheese and ¼ cup of the real deal (e.g., mozzarella + pecorino) when you want the flavor of the real thing (because cheese = heaven) but the volume of something a little lighter on the arteries.

#protip

One fast food that's A-OK with me? Pizza. Veggie pizza with extra veggies (of course!) is a good option when you're in a bind—as long as you can purchase it by the slice. Order a slice of veggie pizza, ask for extra veggies on the slice if that's available, or start with a house or side salad. That'll drive the fiber content up, which will help you stay satisfied and keep that delicious cheesy flavor. I love pizza because it's a nutrient-dense choice when prepared the right way: carbs from the dough; protein from the cheese; and fiber, plus vitamins and minerals from tomatoes. It's just that since pizza usually lacks a little on the veggie front, we find ourselves elbow-deep in dough and feeling like we want *more*. Veggies are your secret weapon—in any meal situation—if you can double up on these, you can have your pizza and eat it, too.

I Don't Eat 'Til Noon Because I'm "Intermittent Fasting"

One popular diet promotes alternating "fasting days," or "periods of fasting" where you go without eating for anywhere between eight and twenty-four hours. Some types of intermittent fasts limit food to a few hours per day, while others limit it to a few days of the week (*brutal, IMO!*). When you're not fasting, you can, for the most part, eat whatever you want (some types of intermittent fasts are "ketogenic," which we'll discuss at length in a few, while others inspire more of a "#cheatday" scenario).

This fasting gives your vital organs, digestive and absorptive hormones, and metabolic functions a "break," and some small studies have, in this set of circumstances, linked the reduction in insulin production and glucose uptake by your fat cells to reducing risk of chronic disease—most promisingly, reducing the incidence of Alzheimer's disease in at-risk populations. The state of "ketosis," in which fat is used for energy (instead of sugar in the form of glucose), occurs when an average adult remains in the fasted state for more than twelve hours (this can also happen on low-carb diets) and has been linked to having a positive health effect.

Overall, the scientific basis for research into the effect of intermittent fasting on disease (known in literature as "biologic plausibility") is that the decreased impact on your fat cells (the ones responsible for the uptake of sugar and fat storage when you eat more than you use) leads to fewer advanced glycation end products (AGEs)—prooxidative compounds associated with increased risk of chronic disease—in the body.

Sure, there's plenty of solid evidence to back up the intermittent fasting craze—it's definitely not all nonsense! But if you do one or more of the following things in the course of a day, intermittent fasting may not be the best option for you:

- *Work for a living*
- Like to read to keep up with the news or for pleasure (it's tough to read *anything* if your blood sugar drops low enough to temporarily blind you)
- Enjoy any form of light exercise (yes, walking to the fridge and having sex count)
- Are responsible for staying awake in any given situation

For the everyday human, there's nothing realistic about intermittent fasting. Having a full day in between fasts in which you can eat absolutely anything can backfire in a big way. It can make you nauseous and dehydrated and also cause weight gain—especially in the long-term, since periods of fasting can decrease your metabolism over time.

While I don't disagree it sounds glorious to eat burgers and sundaes only on certain days of the week (and abstain from food entirely on others), this type of decision-making puts you at two extreme, opposing "sides" of metabolic balance right now! Plus, you can actually achieve the same benefits with a little schedule shifting. Research has found that eating an earlier dinner (and cutting off the grazing afterward) can also initiate ketosis—especially if you're inclined to sleep in the next day. Experiment with eating an early bird special dinner (6 p.m. at the latest!), closing the kitchen afterward, and not eating again until you sit down for a full breakfast around 8 a.m. the following day.

Right-Now Rule #3: Stay Accountable

Sometimes accountability can simply mean staying accountable *to yourself* and your goal of how you want to feel. Yes, *feel*. Not just how you want to look right now, or how healthy you want to be in twenty-five years. Sometimes, being accountable is as simple as following through on the things you say you want to do. Case in point: You want to work out in the mornings, but you always sleep through the available time. You want to "eat better this year," but you just bought yourself a deep fryer. And so on.

In order to help you personalize an eating plan, you're going to have to write down what you eat. Yes, I know, the food log is a total drag, but it's going to evolve into a good thing. (Quickly!)

1. **Write down what you eat**—for just three days—and be honest with yourself, please! We've all done it: record "I only had a rice cake and some tea today!" even as we're trying to clean the take-out food stain off the page. This is for the sake of ultimately knowing how, when, and why you eat, and simply *taking notice of your own eating habits.* You can even keep track in the form of emails to yourself— shoot yourself an email from your phone about what you ate in your last meal. Any time you pick at the granola in the office? Email a note to yourself. Having cocktail peanuts during happy hour and you suddenly don't know *where they went*? Take a pic, save it as your background, and remind yourself that you owe this bar a jar of Virginia Cocktail peanuts. (*Just kidding!*) But seriously: Screenshots and photos are the easiest way to keep a record of what went down at any given meal or snack, so you can do this in the moment before you dig in (*unless you're a food blogger, in which case, keep garnishing!*).

    Tons of research have shown that people who stay accountable to *someone* or *something* (e.g., a friend, a schedule, an exercise class) are much more likely to make long-term changes that stick—because that *person* or *thing* is always there to help the person stay on track. Doesn't sound much like rocket science, right? It's not. In fact, studies indicate that simply the act of writing things down (what you're eating, your weekly exercise class schedule) can help you create a habit because you've literally put it out into the world as a veritable "announcement."

2. **Know what it will look like!** Your next tool for not skipping meals? Know what you're generally in the mood for, and make these options available to you by keeping them top of mind. On your commute to the office, you're going to think of one to three meals that are *readily accessible to you* from your office or that you can have delivered to

you, and think about what you're usually in the mood to eat around noon. Then make sure you have a healthful snack nearby that will scratch the itch without blowing up your goals while you're waiting to pick up or receive your meal. This is another good way to avoid making snap or panicked decisions about food that aren't going to support your health-promoting plans.

3. **Schedule.** Actually schedule meals and snacks in your calendar and set it so you'll get that little "Reminder" notification one hour before. That's also an easy aid to keep you accountable to doing *what you said you were going to do*, which was *not* skipping meals. (*Outlook, for the win!*)

4. **Have a plan B.** What if you encounter a scheduling emergency during the time you were supposed to pick up your soup from Hale and Hearty? You'll need to have something on hand to tide you over. This should be filling enough to get you through *dealing with the emergency*, but not so filling that you fall asleep after eating it. It should also be nonperishable, so that you can buy it today and keep it around in a drawer for as long as you need to.

#protip

In food safety, we consider the "danger zone" to be a temperature range between 41 and 140 degrees. Bacteria in perishable food begins to grow quickly (in as little as twenty minutes) when the food is left unrefrigerated. Never leave food out more than two hours. Eating food in which the bacteria growth has reached dangerous levels can make you sick.

The Satiety Scale

This is the meat of why you've kept that ~~soul-crushing~~ handy food journal: You're about to change your perception of "hunger" and fullness. Think of your appetite on a scale of 1 to 10. Number 1 is that feeling where if you don't eat something *right now*, you're probably going to start gnawing on your computer mouse. Number 10, by contrast, is that feeling you get after Thanksgiving that there might be an actual *whole bird* (and perhaps two types of pie) in your belly.

Your new goal is to eat every three to four hours and to write down how hungry you are before and after you eat. The goal for practicing purposes is to be at a 3 or 4 on the scale before you eat and at around 6 (aim for a max of 8) after you eat. It's okay to eat until you feel stuffed while you're practicing this—in fact, that's a good thing! It means you're learning something about yourself, and *what food and how much food* made you feel too full. Eventually that strategy will actually turn into something that happens instinctively, rather than something you have to write down—but give yourself time.

"I Feel Physically Full, but I'm Not Satisfied—I Still Want Something Else!"

The reason I do the satiety scale exercise with clients is because so many of us suffer from this *epidemic* of what I like to call the "full-but-not-satisfied syndrome" (FNSS). You've experienced this, I'm sure: In people on "low-fat diets," FNSS occurs after eating things like a bowl of pasta with tomato sauce, then thinking, *OMG, why am I still hungry?!* (*There was no protein in your bowl of starch, Sally!*) In people on "low-carb" diets, it occurs after having steak for dinner and then thinking, *I just ate an* actual cow, *and I am dying to eat another.* (*Chill, Dougie—you needed some vegetables. Have a sweet potato!*)

FNSS is a major "trigger" point for many of us in our relationships with overeating or that feeling of "blowing it." The more we can identify when we are feeling FNSS, the more we'll be able to start identifying which foods leave us wanting more and which foods actually let us leave a meal ready to move on with life and not think about eating again for a few hours. (*But no more than four, K?*)

"Seconds" Decision Tree

You're postdinner, and you want to nosh your face off. But before you do, give yourself a beat by having a look at this handy decision tree for determining when you really want more and when you really have other factors at play. Your goal is to rule out whether you (a) are really thirsty instead of hungry, (b) are full without actually feeling all that satisfied, or (c) just need a little something else before bed. (I mean, *don't we have two stomachs and one is for dessert?!*)

- **Rule out thirst:** 16 oz H_2O, seltzer, or unsweetened tea/coffee flavored as you normally would
- Even if you're not feeling completely parched, have a cup or two (8–16 oz) of water, seltzer, or a hot bev like tea or coffee. It'll help you decide what's next if you can at least rule out that what you're actually craving is simple hydration

- **Rule out *legit* hunger:**
- Did your exercise schedule change? Did you skip any meals today? How big was your breakfast? Know where you are so you can hack your habits for next time. Now, assess where you are on the satiety scale:
- 4–5: go for "seconds" of a meal
- 5–7: but you still need a little something: 1 oz chocolate or any single-serve treat

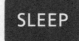

- **Rule out exhaustion** (aka, GO TO BED):
- Are you sure you're not just exhausted? Start counting sheep. Sweet dreams!

Did you skip any meals today?

Did you work out today, or did you put in more than your average day of physical activity? If the answer is yes, have a snack.

Are you having a case of feelings (aka you're bored, sad, lonely, happy, or celebrating something) and thus want to eat more, even if you don't actually feel hungry?

Is there something else you would prefer to be doing besides eating right now? (And, um…is it within the scope of reasonable social/professional code of conduct to actually go and do *that*…? If so, by all means, do that instead!)

But First, Water

Even if you're not feeling completely parched, have a cup or two (8 to 16 ounces) of water, seltzer, or a hot beverage like tea or coffee. It'll help you decide what's next if you can at least rule out that what you're actually craving is simple hydration.

Determine Where You Are on the Satiety Scale

If it's hovering around a 4 or a 5, go for more of a veggie-heavy combo of food (like an extra scoop of stir-fry; leftovers of the salad you made yesterday, etc.). If you're lower than a 4, make sure there's a little protein in there, too (like an egg, or some chicken, fish, or beans so that you're not feeling hunger pangs again in a half hour). If it's hovering around 5 to 7 but you still feel like eating—→ Did you skip any meals today? Are you craving something sweet/savory? If it's savory, try a veg-heavy snack; if it's sweet, have 1- to 1.5-ounce pieces of chocolate, which should be at the ready in the pantry or freezer: around five Hershey's Kisses, two pieces of Ghirardelli, around five Dove chocolate squares, one mini Magnum or Klondike Bar, or a pack of Dole Dippers.

Are You Sure You're Not Just Tired?

Every time you eat is a chance to practice changing your strategy and building confidence in your own eating habits and ability to navigate your schedule. So go to bed! Tomorrow's a new day—let it go, count some sheep, and dream about breakfast tomorrow. (Night night!)

3

I Don't Have Any Time
(or Funds!) for "Wellness"

After this chapter, you will...

- clarify pervasive "wellness" myths that are stagnating your progress;
- curate your preventative health habits based on your personal schedule, time, and resources; and
- learn to identify aspirational content versus attainable ideas that will work for *you*.

When "Wellness" Works for You

Your exposure to the wellness world is a somewhat less obvious aspect of the info jungle. Not only are you hearing about wellness from all sides of the media, but you're also likely exposed in other ways: Food and fitness news-feeds deliver their goods to your phone (or other device) via social media, including Facebook, Twitter, Pinterest, Snapchat, and Instagram. These are vehicles that enable us to learn new things, but they also expose us to lots of new myths, half-truths, and sound-bite science that make it *even harder* to discern what might benefit us versus what will be more of a vacuum of our time, money, and mental and emotional effort.

Every new thing you try, every new recipe you experiment with, and every new ideology you internalize should be aimed at one or both of the following things:

- *Helping* you make sure that more of your meals and snacks are produce-based (that means vegetables or fruits, people).
- *Helping* you to move your tush, aka stay physically active *more often*.

It's that simple. When it comes to food and health, if the advice being given to you will help you eat more real, whole vegetables and fruit (notice that I didn't say "drink"), or will get you off your couch and outside for a walk (even if it's just around the damn block!), and the site, social media feed, or person who is distributing said knowledge gets you to take these actions *without making you feel bad about yourself*, then this advice is *working* for you.

In this chapter, we're going to look at what the world of wellness is, talk about how to discern who's real and who's just selling something, and explore three ways to manage the influx of "wellness" content to make it actually useful in achieving our goals.

Translating Aspirational Content into Attainable Practices

We come from a variety of different backgrounds, ranging in various levels of confidence related to the vast black hole that is information concerning "wellness" (aka doing things in the name of taking care of ourselves). But in this day and age, I think it's safe to assume two things about you as a reader of this book:

1. You feel pressed for time—all of the time—and you believe that making a health-related change would require cloning yourself in order to actually get it done.
2. You feel like a real commitment to your health means a commitment to spending most of your paycheck on food and/or fitness—regardless of how much money you make.

Yep. We *all* feel this way.

So let's sort through the data a little bit and start making some distinctions about the sources we should take seriously versus the sources we should just keep scrolling through.

Requiring Effort = Aspirational; Resourcefulness = Inspirational

There's a difference between things that are aspirational and things that are inspirational. Think back to chapter 1, when we first introduced the concept of trying things that are 80 percent attainable and 20 percent aspirational. Social media have this annoying tendency of tricking you into thinking that 100 percent of all things deemed "wellness" have to be aspirational in order to be *beneficial for you*, a form of "all-or-nothing thinking" (which is a TDT, but you knew that already). But that mind-set can lead to a fast burnout and make you want to give up altogether.

RULE OF THUMB

Aspirational "content" should be taken at face value and used as inspiration for your personal ideas, interests, and inspiration related to your personal health and self-care practices. Following this rule of thumb and thinking of social media as an accountability tool can help you change an out-of-your-comfort-zone activity into a new choice that over time becomes a habit (and is naturally integrated into the whole 80 percent attainable piece of your lifestyle).

Information Metabolism

A casual scroll through social media feeds can be the single greatest trigger to making us feel like we're not *enough*. Of course, we *know* that everyone has problems and that social media is a hyperedited sizzle reel of life's highlights. But we may be a little less *tuned in to* how we actually internalize messages that are fed to us by our social feeds and allow them, unknowingly, to change our inner monologues as we scroll.

Let's say your favorite food blogger posts a picture of a gloriously green and pink Lilly Pulitzer–esque smoothie bowl on Instagram. It is *THE* poster child for #wellness. In fact, you're certain that if you looked up "healthy" in the dictionary, you'd find this gloriously Pantone-perfect mint-and-flamingo-colored bowl with three errant blackberries strewn by the side of the bowl and a crescent moon of chia seeds sprinkled on top with some type of sprig or shrub in the middle. (*Food bloggers on social media love a good garnish, no?!*)

So, of course, after seeing this yummy and beautiful smoothie bowl, you're excited to try re-creating it for yourself. But when the results of what you create in your kitchen don't even hold a candle to this professionally styled and photographed bowl, you may start to feel a little prickle of unworthiness as something similar to this thought enters your mind: *That person is better at life than I am.*

If you're reading this and thinking, *I definitely don't ever think that—this clearly has nothing to do with me!* well, that's great for *you*, Tommy, but for many of us such a situation can be the beginning of a wellness-induced shame spiral that might sound something like this:

I love this blog; that smoothie bowl looks so ahhh-mazing! Let's see what's in it: OMG, pitaya! Red dragon fruit is so trendy right now; I wonder if it's a "superfood." Oh, and there's coconut oil in there, because of course. And there's #kale in here! The blogger says she used two bunches of kale, which seems like so much and honestly there must be something wrong with me because everyone loves it but it kinda tastes like dirt to me. How are those berries so perfectly round? I bought frozen cherries last week and they looked like bright red clumps of glacier when I took them out of the package! I wonder how she gets such perfect freezer frost!? I'm pretty certain mine were just freezer-burned. Oh, and are those hemp seeds, chia seeds, or flaxseeds? WHAT?! She says they're ACORN FLOUR. I don't know, can humans even *eat* acorns? The caption says it has a lot of "vegan minerals that boost vitality," so I guess that means yes (or it explains why squirrels can run so fast). Wait, can *minerals* even be vegan or not vegan? Where do you even *buy* acorn flour?!

"Clean" sounds about as life-changing as "detox," but I'm of the faith that the word is best used in reference to household disinfectants and laundry detergent. #Cleaneating (and its cousin, #eatclean) is one of those terms that gets tossed around left and right among bloggers, influencers, and even food companies and manufacturers. But does it have a real definition? Nope.

Nada! Zip. Zero! The original philosophy appears to be one I think we could all get on board with: more plants, whole grains, carefully sourced animal- and plant-based protein, plus nuts, seeds, and oils. Personally, what I used to like about the general concept is that it seemed to promote an eating style that minimized highly processed foods and pushed for ones that were as close to nature as possible. But these days (and especially in the context of social media mayhem!) I'm worried that #cleaneating has become a shell of its former nutrient-dense self. What was once a sense of awareness about food seems to have spiraled into a diet culture–driven caste system. Not only does the phrase establish a hierarchical model for eating healthily, but also it's yet another medium for body- and food-shaming—especially because much of what you'll see in these posts is promoting products that ultimately require some underlying behaviors that are antithetical to keeping you on track with what works for you by often promoting elimination-based eating habits and attribution of value (good or bad) to certain foods in isolation of what else you eat every day! So my advice: Ignore posts with this tag. No one has the time, emotional bandwidth, or financial resources to worry about the exclusivity and restriction of this distant cousin of "detox"!

We've all done something similar—I'd be hard-pressed to find some- one who *hasn't*. Social media dieting information and advice don't have the structure or support you need to make lasting change in your life. Social media can be great with arm's-length viewership, and you might pick up a tidbit or two of helpful info. If you're feeling a little isolated on your journey to better health, the camaraderie can encourage you and help you keep focused. But if you're serious about the changes you want to make, then you need to find what works for you personally—not a #squad of food bloggers!

How do you find what works for you while limiting exposure to shame- inducing information? Here are some tips.

It's Not About You: What to Notice Without Judgment

I had a dance teacher in college who used this phrase often as it relates to *movement through space*: "Notice, but don't judge."

(*Don't you just love that?!*)

The idea behind the phrase is that you can notice things about the way your classmates dance and the way *you* dance without ascribing any particular *value* to it—and be extra aware of the fact that it's our tendency to do the former instead of the latter. The point of noticing without judging is to take in information without applying it to yourself and your own sense of worth. The same theory can be applied to the way you *notice* behaviors on social media without instinctively making them something that has to have *meaning or value to you.*

The tendency these days is to metabolize social media and other sources of wellness content. You're digesting and absorbing content regardless of where it comes from or how relevant it is to your life. Your brain, much like your liver if you'll recall, is repackaging and reusing this information in ways you're not necessarily fully aware of 100 percent of the time.

Asking you to notice but not judge may sound a bit like asking you to rise to become some seriously evolved meditation guru, but what's crucial in improving your state of health is to do so in ways that actually work for you, and that requires filtering the information you take in.

Allow me to illustrate this with a professional example. If you were to review the accounts that my RD colleagues and I "follow," you'd see many that don't necessarily align with evidence-backed scientific consensus about nutrition and preventive health. But we're always checking out Instagram stories and looking for trending, nutrition-related tags, ~~accidentally~~ double-tapping on photos of people we may or may not have ever met.

(*Don't we all do that?!*)

It's important for me as a dietitian to stay informed so that I can help clients, readers, family, and friends discern the beneficial info from the not-so-great stuff and make better choices. I try to stay in the know as much as possible about what's "out there," and I also stay up-to-date on new scientific studies and developing areas of health and food research. Doing *both* of these helps me to identify trends and understand how science (and sometimes, lack thereof!) is communicated to better help others find what works best for them—I'm noticing without personalizing or internalizing—from a place of professional curiosity. And to that end, I'd encourage you to do the same! What if it was your *actual job to notice without judgment*? You might feel a little more removed (and less affected!) by all of that *noise*.

Acacia is an FDA-approved emulsifier that's sustainably sourced from Nairobi. You'll find it used as a sugar substitute in yogurt, ice cream, and coffee creamer products, marketed as a healthier version of another emulsifier called *carrageenan*. Both are safe, but acacia is more fun to say!

Here's an exercise on how to filter your information intake:

Step 1: Identify the social media accounts and websites you don't want to avoid entirely, which would most likely include
- your relatives and friends;
- your workplace colleagues and superiors; and
- sources of information that provide you with an edge in a specific area of your life.

Step 2: Identify *why* you don't want to avoid them.

Step 3: Write that sh*t down.

Step 4: Now review all the other accounts you follow and sites you frequent. If this person or the information provided is either (a) not all that significant to you personally or professionally in the big scheme of things, or (b) making you feel more crappy and powerless than happy, informed, and empowered, then consciously make the decision to tap Unfollow and do it ASAP.

Step 5: Remember that we have enough psychological stressors in our everyday lives that knowingly or unknowingly make us feel bad about ourselves. So, for the last time: Do you really need to *keep following* the #fitnessinfluencer who is constantly posting bikini pics from a different beautiful beach every week? (Maybe; that's *your* call—not mine. I just wanted to check in *one last time to make 100 percent sure!*) I'm asking you to respect the difference between knowing certain details about a topic or person, and using that information to inform you in a different, more useful way. It's not manipulative; it's informed. And most of all, it's resourceful!

Conscious Unfollowing: What to Ignore

Information sources to beware of tout "wellness" practices that have one or all of the following traits: They're expensive; there doesn't appear to be much (if any) science to back up their benefits; they conflate consensus-based science with controversy-based science; they misuse terminology; there is evidence that they're harmful; or there's no evidence that they're harmful, but they don't appear to be necessary. This takes a kind of conscious unfollowing (to borrow some inspiration from an impactful wellness "guru" . . .).

Anything or Anyone Who Promotes a Product with a Health "Promise"

There's a time-honored saying that goes a little something like this: "The only thing that's guaranteed in life is that there are no guarantees." Well, my friends: This, too, applies to how scientists feel about science. If a product is making promises or guarantees or if it is using the word *proven*, please abort mission! If you work in any peer-reviewed area of study, you are *hyper*conscious of these words, because it's rare to find a specific, direct link in terms of one product and a direct health outcome (see chapter 1 for a refresher on association versus causation!).

With that in mind, sponsored content can be highly valuable and introduce you to some really great products that might introduce you to other things you come to love. (*Kombucha? Matcha? OAT MILK?! Cool!*) But where you can get into trouble is when these items promise something that is outside the realm of biological plausibility. Or conversely, it's within the realm of biological plausibility, but making claims of any kind that overpromise and possibly underdeliver. And unless the person you're following is a scientist whom you trust to have led the independent research affirming that the product really does what it claims to do (*Now, THAT is an Instagram account I would follow! Why aren't there more scientists on social media, honestly?! #scinflu encer? Let's make it a thing!*), you're much better off eating real food and moving your tush regularly rather than double-tapping on a health "promise" or promotional benefit.

"Clean Eating"

This phrase and the hashtags #cleaneating and #eatclean have spread like wildfire—which is, quite frankly, amazing to me given that there is no real definition of the term! The piece of this (#clean, #vegan, #glutenfree) pie I dislike the most is that it disregards the lack of access—as well as a lack of time and money—that many of us face when it comes to finding perfect, farmer's market–fresh food. Frankly, it's elitist. For a lot of people, clean eating is simply code for attempting to be thin (above all else), green-juice-loving, yoga-practicing perfect pictures of health.

So ask yourself: Is the post, article, product, or person touting some philosophy making it more inspiring, helpful, easy, and fun for me to *eat more produce* or *move my tushy*? If the answer is yes, then okay—keep it. But if the post, article, product, or person makes you feel guilty about what you packed for lunch, or makes a healthful lifestyle seem so strict that you just want to give up and get some fast food, it's time to #unfollow.

Dietary Supplements and Weight-Loss Pill Companies (...and Their #Influencers)

Real talk: You don't need these, unless you take them under the supervision of a medical professional who says you do need them for a highly specific reason. Some good examples: People who don't eat fish or any type of seafood, ever, may need some choline, DHA/EPA, and vitamin D; people who don't get outside all that much (or are clinically deficient in vitamin D) will need some cholecalciferol (the fancy name for that vitamin!) with calcium (which optimizes absorption in your GI tract); women who are pregnant, who want to be pregnant, or who are lactating may opt in on prenatal vitamins; people who have caught a stomach bug and are now having trouble with regularity might try a probiotic supplement.

If you're thinking, *So what?! If there's no harm in taking supplements, then I should try it!* Well…chew on this: Dietary supplements aren't overseen by the FDA, meaning they're not evaluated for safety and efficacy in the same way that food and medications are before they're available for purchase on the market—so you may not be getting *exactly* what you believe you're paying for. And if you are? Well, regardless of evaluation, certain nutrients, when consumed in supplement form rather than food form, can have unintended effects. One (rather dramatic) example of that is prooxidation, a side effect of antioxidant supplementation, meaning they induce oxidative stress rather than lessening it. That can cause more harm than good to your organ tissues (*which is likely what you were trying to minimize, right,*

Sandy?!) and increase your risk of chronic disease, including heart disease and some cancers.

Most of All: People, Websites, and Blogs That, Often for No Real Reason at All, Make You Feel Bad About Yourself

These are the people and information sources that have found their way into your feed and stayed well past their welcome—not *necessarily* because you're so keen on beating yourself up before you get out of bed in the morning or because you relish feeling sorry for yourself. (*Yet they seem to lead you down that gut-wrenching road anyway!*) Take five minutes daily to go through each of your social media networks or email newsletters and "unfollow," "block from newsfeed," or "unsubscribe" from the folks and sources that you can't just unsee. Life is really just too damn short for low-dose, consistent hits of emotional stress delivered to you via newsfeed.

(*Seriously, @cleaneatsandbikinitweets, you're just NOT helping!*)

The Superfraud of "Superfoods"

File under "Meaningless Terms That Are *Everywhere*": Superfood is top of that list, though in contrast to "clean eating," it's actually *defined* by *Merriam-Webster*, but the definition is one that leaves all of us in the field of nutrition science feeling just a tad befuddled: "a food (such as salmon, broccoli, or blueberries) that is rich in compounds (such as antioxidants, fiber, or fatty acids) considered beneficial to a person's health."

While it's true that the foods listed by *M-W* are tops in terms of nutrient density, the gripe I have with calling any food in isolation "super" is that no one is achieving any type of miracle health status from having a serving of broccoli in a diet otherwise riddled with chocolate-chip-cookie cream puffs, right? Foods are only as "super" for you as the context and consistency with which you're adding more nutritious options to meals and snacks. Health benefits can be subjective and overblown when taken out of context—I mean, if you're just eating broccoli at every meal, that can be risky, too! If the dose makes the poison, then surely Paracelsus would have a field day with this one.

With this in mind, let's discuss a more expansive list of foods with the attributes *M-W* lists: fiber, antioxidants, and essential fatty acids.

- **Plant-based foods that are in their whole-food form (aka, ones you can actually chew):** All foods you can chew are "super," but in particular, any vegetable or fruit; any legume and pulse crop, like chickpeas, lentils, beans, and peas; nuts and seeds; 100 percent whole grains; plant-based (fruit-, vegetable-, nut-, seed-, or legume-based oils, or any mix of those when used for cooking purposes). Plants in whole-food form provide the optimal nutrient composition for both short-term and long-term health and weight management, and a lot of that is thanks to fiber and a variety of antioxidant properties. Based on this new knowledge: Another top source of chewable superness is:

- **Plant-based ingredients with which you cook or caffeinate (in their simplest form):** Spices and herbs can also have tons of "super" properties, but across the literature we find that a lot of the more promising studies are the ones looking at association (population) studies, meaning that their benefits are also better illustrated in the context of dietary patterns (e.g., plant-based foods you can actually chew), not when extracted, isolated, and crushed into a powder or pill. Similarly, plants that become other food ingredients that are drinkable and worthwhile: tea and coffee (when consumed in their plain, unsweetened form!).

- **Plant-based ingredients that serve as fuel for animal (especially *marine*) protein sources you eat:** Seafood is across-the-board "super" (there are some select exceptions—we'll cover those later on!). But the main reason for that is the type of plants. Lots of seaweed, lots of kelp, and lots of algae. (YUM!)

The "super" way to *eat food* is in its intended state, aka chewable (versus drinkable); raw or cooked (depending on type and meal occasion); and using some plant-based oils (dietary fat helps fat-soluble vitamins found in plants to digest and absorb more efficiently in your GI tract). Since plants positively *rule*, eat more of those, more regularly, and you'll be even more *super* than you already are.

(*I didn't think that was even possible!*)

#protip

Skip the Berry Bowl

Açai, pitaya, and any blends, bowls, or smoothie kits are often made with fruit juice concentrate or fruit concentrate and/or fruit puree. While the FDA allows this form of sweetness to be added to foods and beverages using the claim "no added sugar," your best bet is easily found fresh whole berries: raspberries, blueberries, blackberries, strawberries—you name it—and reaping the benefits of about 8 grams of fiber and only 60 calories per cup. Real food sources of fiber are satiety-boosting and heart-healthy and have a negligible impact on your glycemic response as compared to the concentrated form (aka smoothie bowls).

Bottom line: The net is *wide* when it comes to all foods deemed "super."

Next, let's unpack some of those claims on food products and nutrients that we see everywhere.

Apple Cider Vinegar

Made from the addition of bacterial cultures and yeast to apple juice, this sweet-tasting fruit vinegar gets some serious hype for reversing everything from diabetes to weight gain. (Quick question: If that were true, wouldn't we all be swilling apple cider vinegar by now?!)

I drink it first thing in the morning. I heard it helps you eat less during the day.

The delayed gastric emptying that's been seen in the (limited) existing research on vinegar is likely caused by the slower rate of digestive enzyme activity in the GI tract, and/or interference with stomach motility, which slows down the rate at which food moves through your stomach to your intestine, making you feel fuller longer. But drinking apple cider vinegar on an empty stomach can be tough on your GI tract long-term and can induce heartburn in those who are prone to it in the short-term. Plus, the feelings of satiety are likely a result of the fact that your entire esophagus is now on fire. Thanks, #wellness!

Does it help to digest carbs?

Sorry, but apple cider vinegar isn't exactly a Kälteen bar (*Mean Girls*, anyone?). One small study linked apple cider vinegar to a lightening of the blood sugar effect of high-carb, high-glycemic-index meals as compared to meals of the same calorie and carb levels, only made with unprocessed, high-fiber carbs. But the results of the study only demonstrated blood sugar–lowering effects of vinegar when consumed with that specific type of carb—aka the ones you're limiting anyway!

And to that end: Flavonoids, an antioxidant compound found in apples, is great for health, but the amount of antioxidants you're *actually* getting in a spoonful of apple cider vinegar is unclear. *Plus, do you really want to live your life drinking a fermented condiment when you could just eat a Honeycrisp and move on?!* Reminder: ACV is a dressing, not a drink.

It's antibacterial, though, right?

Nope. Simply because an "acid" is a by-product of vinegar production doesn't mean vinegar is a germ-killer—nor does it "detox" any vital organs (c'mon—you *know this*!). Adding vinegar can help during food prep, but not in killing bacteria, viruses, or anything else you contracted during your #wellnessretreat in the desert!

While I wish this were the potion marketing makes it out to be, one tablespoon, shot glass, or bucket of vinegar in the morning *will not help with weight loss*! The only research to date that has shown any link to weight loss was poorly controlled and conducted with a tiny sample size. Plus, subjects in the study were put on a lower-calorie diet to begin with!

Listen up: There's one thing I really *love* about apple cider vinegar (and you probably already know where I'm headed with this): You can use it as part of a salad dressing—*yes, in the salad bowl, not on the side*— as a flavor enhancer. Vinegar has zero calories and can be used *liberally* without much of a health risk (but GERD-sufferers: Consider yourself warned!). If you're sipping the stuff solely for its purported health "benefits," though, science says you're a little out of luck (at least for now). Your best bet is to fill up on plant-based foods, which will provide all the benefits you need to stay sated. Bottom line: Vinegar is best used in salads, not supplements.

Collagen

There's nothing in human studies that has supported the use of collagen so far. What I like about it, however, is that some companies (like Vital Proteins) are making some portable versions, which is cool if you want to make a more filling beverage (a homemade smoothie) by including protein powder. The same idea applies to coffee—but not for any "bulletproof" something-or-other.

But do you *need collagen*? Nope. Claims of its benefits include terms such as *antiaging, elasticity-promoting, anti-inflammatory*, you name it. You'll see collagen on broth and stock labels, which is actually where it belongs (there's protein and calcium in "bone broths" because of the actual *animal bones*). You can eat collagen in the form of an egg, steak, fish, chicken, turkey, or cheese. Collagen is a type of protein, and therefore, when we eat protein we're eating collagen. It just sounds sexier to say "collagen" because we associate it with antiaging products, which allow us to put collagen on our *faces*. And while there's some pretty hearty research supporting the theory that if you're deficient in protein or in need of wound healing, your protein needs are higher, the truth is that most Americans are eating about double the recommended daily intake. (Per day, Americans need between 0.8 and 1.0 g of protein per kilogram [2.2 pounds] of body weight.)

A similar comparison? Biotin and B-vitamin supplements, which are also touted among wellness enthusiasts for their "hair-growth-stimulating nutrients" or benefits to your nails, skin, and hair. But to date, there's only limited evidence supporting the idea that this works in reality in the same ways that it works in in vitro (test-tube!) studies.

Bummer, I know!

Coconut Oil

Let's clarify a few things once and for all, shall we?!

Does it burn belly fat?

This is not a thing, people! But a few small-scale studies have linked extra-virgin coconut oil consumption to decreased waist circumference in individuals at risk for heart disease or diabetes—but those with any significant results had already been on a weight-loss diet in the first place! Plus, spot training or "burning" belly fat is a cute way that exceptionally smart people in digital media get *you* to click on an article online. (Hey, no judgment! "Burn Belly Fat with These Coconut Oil–Laden Superfoods" = a stellar-sounding article I'd click on, too!)

I heard it has antibacterial properties, doesn't it?

About half of the fatty acids found in coconut oil are from lauric acid, which has been linked to antimicrobial, antifungal effects that may reduce the risk of certain acute and chronic ailments and diseases (e.g., a yeast infection or type 2 diabetes). But that's no reason to bathe your internal organs in the stuff. Research is still ongoing on the topic, but you would have to consume high amounts of the oil to truly reap its benefits. Dietary fat racks up quickly in the calories-from-saturated-fat department, so it may not be worth the risk. (*Relax, Lisa! Just use some hand sanitizer and you'll be just fine this winter!*)

But coconut oil definitely revs metabolism and helps you lose weight, right?

Alas, in our dreams. The only truly variable factor in changing your metabolic rate significantly is to increase the ratio of your lean body mass to your free fat mass (in other words: More muscles = increased metabolism). While some foods high in certain compounds (like caffeine, capsaicin, and catechins) may contribute to a *mild* and *temporary increase* in metabolism, coconut oil has yet to produce any real verified results on that front.

My aunt forwarded an article to me that says coconut oil is heart-healthy.

Nope. But there's no 100 percent guarantee it will *seal your fate* for heart disease, either.

The stats: One tablespoon of coconut oil provides more than half the amount of saturated fat that both the 2015–2020 USDA *Dietary Guidelines for Americans* and the American Heart Association recommend *per day*! Foods that are high in saturated fat *have* been linked to an increase in total cholesterol in addition to an increase in LDL (otherwise known as "bad" cholesterol). In some studies, coconut oil helped to raise HDL ("good" cholesterol) and total cholesterol—without necessarily affecting LDL. But these indications are not enough to make a recommendation across the board. Since other heart-healthy oils, like soybean, hemp seed, extra-virgin olive oil, and rapeseed (aka canola), have been linked to lowering LDL *and* total cholesterol overall (they provide plant sterols and polyphenolic compounds that are also linked to decreasing heart disease risk), these options are still better alternatives for those at risk for heart disease.

Okay, fine—but its smoke point is higher than that of other oils, right?

The truth: At around 350 degrees, coconut oil has a relatively *low* smoke point as compared to other plant-based, antioxidant-packed oils, such as corn, canola, grapeseed, sesame seed, avocado, peanut, and soybean. Actually, its smoke point is only 30 degrees higher than that of extra-virgin olive oil. While it's nutritionally similar to butter, it may be a better alternative to shortening for vegans or those who are severely lactose-intolerant. Check labels on any plant-based oil that's solid at room temperature—that's a clear indicator of hydrogenation, which can have negative effects on your cholesterol and long-term heart health.

Everybody says that coffee plus coconut oil helps you lose weight.

Let's answer this one by looking at this in context for a minute. Coffee with coconut oil could, theoretically, make you gain weight if you're consuming a lot of it *regularly,* since it's higher in calories than if you'd just had a skim latte and called it a day. Plus, when you consider how it might be prepared given the combo of ingredients (*and we both know you have a heavy hand with that coconut oil, Clarissa!*), *how* you make it determines how big of an impact it'll have on your day: 135 to 470 calories, up to 47 grams of saturated fat (over 200 percent of the recommended daily intake), and zero grams of protein. A better bet: Drink coffee and tea black, without added sweetener, or consider making it a conscious, protein-packed source of calories at breakfast: A 16-ounce nonfat or skim latte can provide up to 13 grams of protein per a 120-calorie serving, which can help tide you over between breakfast and lunch (and is better for keeping your metabolism going throughout the day. And while all things "bulletproof" sound sexy as hell, I wish they did any of the things they typically promote (especially that whole "cognitive boost" claim—I'd have slathered coconut oil on my chemistry flash cards *years ago!*).

On the flip side: If you really feel like consuming this many calories in beverage form is keeping you satisfied throughout the morning (*it always comes back to where you're at on the satiety scale, people!*), it may have *some* promise. Coconut oil's polyphenolic compounds (aka plant-based antioxidants) may help to prevent a key protein in Alzheimer's disease from doing its dirty work. That said, most other plant-based oils have been linked to decreasing dementia risk, cognitive decline, and neurodegenerative disease for the same reason. Bottom line: If you love the *taste* of coconut oil, use it (and butter) when cooking. Opt to use *more* of the other plant-based oils for your day-to-day culinary needs.

Choose coconut oil occasionally for flavor, but mix it up with other types of plant-based oils and butter for your day-to-day culinary needs!

Probiotics

Fermented seasonings, drinks, and foods like miso, kimchi, tempeh, kombucha, and sauerkraut are chock-full of probiotics, beneficial bacteria that can help boost gut health. Since the gut serves as the "bodyguard" of your immune system (everything you eat is filtered through the gut before entering your bloodstream!), loads of research continues to be published with new and significant findings on the crucial importance of eating probiotic-containing foods. While the more processed versions are never ideal (probiotics are being added to everything from sugary beverages to candy!), eating the real, whole-food sources (like the ones mentioned above and unsweetened yogurts with five or more live and active cultures added) is the best way to maintain good gut health habits! An offshoot of the probiotics craze is the low-FODMAP (fermentable oligo-, di-, and monosaccharides and polyols) diet, which refers to the types of natural sugars found in many carbohydrate-based foods that can trigger GI upset due to malabsorption in your small intestine. The diet is recommended for those with IBS (irritable bowel syndrome) or IBD (inflammatory bowel disease, like Crohn's or colitis)—since FODMAPs are in lots of foods, it's certainly not a trend for just anyone to try (and for that matter: It's *not* a weight-loss diet!). There's plenty of research that supports the beneficial effects of low-FODMAP diets for individuals suffering from a whole host of IBS symptoms, so consult a gastroenterologist and seek out an RD for specific recs if you're keen on giving it a go.

Things You Can Take with a Grain of...er, Salt

Sorry for the pun. Here are some ideas on key takeaways from each:

- **Paleo.** The only thing to like about "paleo" diets? They do emphasize real food, although they cut out a lot of food groups for random reasons. (*Did the first humans really not eat peanuts?! Why?!*) Checking in on tags like #paleo can help inspire some main-course recipe ideas.
- **Veganism/Vegetarianism.** Eating more vegetables is always a good idea.
- **Low-Carb.** Looking for low-carb foods can lead you to beneficial high-fiber foods that you might not have tried previously. Super-high-fiber bran crackers (such as GG Scandinavian) are one favorite of low-carb dieters. The range of seeds, nuts, brans, vegetables, and fruits available to satisfy those following a low-carb eating plan is substantial.
- **Dairy-Free.** The great thing about the rise in the popularity of pulse products (since the United Nations General Assembly declared 2016

the International Year of Pulses) is that they can serve as dairy alternatives and are fortified with the same ingredients. Ice creams and ice pops that are vegan are often infinitely worse for you, though, thanks to coconut milk and added sugar, so be sure to look for items that (a) do not have sugar as the first ingredient, and (b) are vegetable- or fruit-based and in a form that you can *chew*.

- **Gluten-Free.** The magic of gluten-free diets is that going without gluten in many scenarios (e.g., there is no gluten-free bread at a given restaurant, so you'll just have to bypass the bread basket and wait for your main course; or there are cupcakes in the break room, but they're not gluten-free, so you'll have to forgo the treat; and so on) means you're also cutting calories from significant and spur-of-the-moment sources.

Products with Supposed "Beauty" Benefits for Your Skin

Examples: spirulina (blue-green algae), aloe water, detox waters, charcoal, clay, and probably pencil lead by the date of this book's publication

Bottom line: There's plenty of research on the benefits of topical products that include ingredients such as aloe and certain vitamins, but as long as your diet contains a good variety of actual foods—you should be good on this front without the algae, charcoal, and so on. Foods that may be linked to healthier skin include nuts, seeds, veggies, and fruit, which have higher amounts of certain polyphenolic compounds that help to protect the skin from damage over time. The jury's still out, though, on extracting any benefit to the skin from a specific nutrient—especially in pill, powder, or juice form.

Adaptogens

Examples: amla, ashwagandha, chlorella, chaga, maca

Bottom line: There's virtually zero science on the actual efficacy of these products, but the concept of adaptogens is legit: Certain properties of these herbs "adapt" to the needs of your body at any given moment in time. And consuming these herbs with their antioxidant properties as seasoning on vegetables has a twofold benefit: It can help you cut back on the amount of sodium you might eat otherwise, and it can help boost the antioxidant properties of the foods you're eating. In research it's pretty difficult to *control* for these types of claims about food products, but using herbs and spices to supplement or in lieu of sodium when you're flavoring your food? That's evidenced-backed *and* delicious!

Supplements That Act as "Sleep" Agents

Examples: melatonin, magnesium

Bottom line: There is some science behind using magnesium and melatonin as sleep agents, but proceed with caution: Magnesium sulfate is also used as a *laxative* (which seems a bit counterintuitive, right? You can't go to sleep if you're on the toilet half the night!). It might be better to simply choose foods with *more magnesium* at bedtime, like a handful of nuts or seeds along with dried, unsweetened dates and figs. Another supplement with some promise in the sleep department is L-arginine. This amino acid is a precursor to nitric oxide, a compound that vasodilates (aka loosens up) blood vessels and is found in dried, unsweetened tart cherries—which will also go nicely with your handful of filberts, aka hazelnuts. (*You're welcome!*)

Snack Before Bed

It'll help you sleep better and go to bed feeling a little bit more sated (being too hungry can keep you up!). Best sleep-inducing combos:

100 Percent Whole-Grain Cereal + Nonfat Milk

While the carbohydrates in cereal help you fall asleep, protein-rich milk helps you stay asleep. How? By eating them together, you'll absorb more of the amino acid tryptophan (usually associated with that post–Thanksgiving meal slump) than you would if you ate them separately. Plus, milk is chock-full of calcium and magnesium, which help you produce melatonin—the hormone responsible for sleep regulation. Just stick to 1 cup of a low-sugar cereal (6 g of sugar or less per serving) with ½ cup of skim milk.

Low-Fat (Plain, Unsweetened!) Greek Yogurt with Melon

Since dehydration can affect your ability to fall and stay asleep, choosing a high-water-volume fruit like melon can make up for any missing drinks during the day. And since melon + dairy products is just a tad reminiscent of "dieting" in the 1980s, you have my blessing to try other fruits, too: apples, oranges, and pears…persimmon, passion fruit, pomegranate (you do you…but all of these are potassium-packed, hydrating options, too!).

Pistachios and Dried Tart Cherries

Pistachios have a winning sleep-inducing combination of protein, vitamin B_6, and magnesium, and dried cherries have been linked to increasing melatonin production, which can help you chill out and get some z's. Aim for about ¼ cup of each so you're not going to bed feeling stuffed.

Cheese and Crackers

Pick a lower-sodium cheese like Emmentaler Swiss to keep salt and saturated fat in check (too much of both can keep you up) and pair it with around 15 small crackers (lower sodium versions = <200 mg so you're not awake all night guzzling H_2O).

Nut Butter and Banana

Bananas and nut butter pack a big vitamin B_6 and magnesium punch, making them ideal for pre-sleep snacking. Stick to a tablespoon of the butter so you're not feeling too full before hitting the hay—another factor that can contribute to a poor night's rest thanks to some (brutal) heartburn. Regardless: Stay upright for about thirty minutes after snacking and before bed. (Great news, because that gives you extra time to keep reading this book! *You're welcome.*)

Decaf Tea and a *Sensible* Biscuit

Okay, stick with me here: I know this sounds a bit like I'm your British great-grandma preaching from a wicker rocking chair "pulpit," but a graham cracker and chamomile combo goes a long way. The tea can hydrate and soothe you (soothing blends = chamomile, cinnamon, and ginger—just read labels so you can check caffeine content). The 100 percent whole grains in a good ol' biscuit, like one or two graham cracker sheets or oat/granola-based "breakfast" bars (like KIND Healthy Grains, Nature Valley, or Kashi) will help you maximize B vitamins and minerals that can help you power down.

Spices That Have Become Supplements

Examples: turmeric, ginger, cinnamon, cloves, garlic

Bottom line: There's a large and growing body of evidence here, but the bioavailability (meaning how much your body can actually absorb) of the pill or powder form of these compounds is virtually nil. For the most part, don't waste your money on these spices/supplements in pill form, but there is some evidence that spice teas (especially peppermint, cinnamon, and ginger) help with GI distress and tummy upset. For seasoning foods, your best bet is to use turmeric and black pepper in the same meal; research has found that the two increase the absorptive properties of certain antioxidants.

Mushroom Beverages

Examples: coffee, tea, and juices

Bottom line: Mushrooms themselves are one of the only plant-based dietary sources of vitamin D, but the real-deal benefits of these veggies is in the fiber they provide in food form only. Eat 'em if you love 'em; skip drinking them in beverages if you don't. The benefits touted by many of the companies who offer mushroom drinks are linked to the coffee or tea in which they're present, but it's not likely you're getting much by way of minerals and antioxidants found in the powdered form.

Anything "Alkaline"

The alkaline diet—also known as the pH eating plan—continues to sport a health halo and attract A-list celebrity endorsers, despite the fact that there is no scientific literature supporting its benefits.

The diet promotes eating foods that are alkaline in chemical composition (like broccoli) *and* foods that are acidic by nature but promote "alkalinity" in your body's cells (such as lemons). The commonality? They're both *produce*. Below, your need-to-know on this gimmick.

Meals and Snacks Can't Actually Change the pH of Your Blood

First things first: Eating any type of "acidic" or "basic" food will not affect your blood pH (measure of acidity and alkalinity). Healthy adults typically have a pH of 7.4—a number considered slightly alkaline, given that 7 is "neutral" on the pH scale of 1 to 14.

Unless your kidneys or lungs are impaired, the acid-base balance of your body doesn't actually move much *at all* one way or the other (and if it did, you wouldn't be here to read this book). So where exactly did this perception come from? Foods can have a temporary impact on cellular mineral content, which determines the "acidity" inside and outside your cells.

If You Have Functioning Vital Organs, Alkaline Foods Are Redundant

In the same vein as "cleanses" that tout their ability to "rest your liver," alkaline diets that claim to give your kidneys a much-needed vacation are equally futile. Properly functioning kidneys are like your body's own filtration system: They help to excrete what you don't need while retaining what you *do* need, thereby regulating your pH level, which fluctuates naturally.

When the ability of your kidneys to "clean" the bloodstream *is* truly impaired, it's often the result of the kidneys being overly taxed by a chronic condition over time—like high blood sugar (uncontrolled diabetes) or high blood pressure (uncontrolled hypertension)—which can both lead to kidney failure. And yes, if these conditions are left untreated, they can cause a change in blood pH (resulting, for example, in a condition called *diabetic ketoacidosis*, which occurs when the body's cells are unable to take in glucose due to either a lack of insulin or long-term insulin-resistance). So while those conditions can be and often are diet-related, their appearance isn't anywhere near as immediate as popular diet fads and of-the-moment medical "experts" have led you to believe.

Bottom line: Alkaline diets do have the benefit of being more plant-based instead of animal-heavy, making them naturally higher in fiber and polyunsaturated fats, and another plus is the limited intake of sodium, sugar, and saturated fat from processed food sources. It's pretty safe to say, however, that the pH of a food isn't the be-all and end-all of what makes it nutritious. In fact, science shows it's got absolutely *nothing* to do with it!

"Alkaline" Is a Synonym for "Smart Marketing"

Alkaline water, usually meaning it has a pH of 9.5 or higher, may taste better to you than regular water, and if that's the case, then by all means, drink up! (HYDRATION FOR ORGAN FUNCTION! may as well be your campaign slogan!) But since an influx of electrolytes—particularly ones that are alkaline—into your GI tract can cause nausea, vomiting, and diarrhea, you might want to go easy on the stuff. Also, alkaline water may have adverse reactions with certain medications, so consult a physician if you drink it regularly.

Bottom line: Sodium bicarbonate, which makes water "alkaline," has been linked to improving lactic acid buildup in athletes, but since the GI side effects are so unpleasant, it's rarely used in practice. Hydrate regularly and often with any type of water you like (fresh, sparkling—you get the point!) and skip waters with alkaline-promoting benefits from synthetic trace minerals.

Anything "Keto"

It's highly possible that you've tried this terrifyingly trendy diet and are *here, with me,* right now as a direct result of a post-ketosis backlash...so in theory, I'm *very* grateful to all things keto! (*I'm kidding!*) But certainly, ketogenic diets have a well-studied benefit—it's just that it happens to be specifically seen in individuals (mostly children) who suffer from epilepsy that's refractory to medication. Here's the deal: In order for your body to stay in ketosis, both carb and protein intake must be limited—a distinct difference from what's commonly known as "modified Atkins" or traditional high-protein, lower-carb diets. That's because high protein intake leads to glucose production through a process called *gluconeogenesis*, which raises blood sugar, stimulates insulin production, and prevents ketosis. In order to rely on dietary fat for most of your calories per day, you've got to be sure you're cutting calories from fiber-rich sources (like fruits, veggies, legumes) and sources rich in lean protein (e.g., fatty fish)—some of the most nutrient-dense foods *on the planet*. If you're eating tons of these foods and claiming to be "keto"? Well, I'd hate to be the bearer of bad news, but you're not really *in a ketogenic state*, Barbara! If you're restricting these foods, counting "net carbs" (a term, still undefined by the FDA, for the total grams of carbohydrates remaining after subtracting the number of fiber grams present in a food), and strictly adhering to keto's parameters, then it's also very likely you're not meeting your micronutrient needs and are likely going to need vitamin and mineral supplementation in pill form. (Recap: We don't always know what's in them, we don't know if they're safe for long-term use, and we don't always know where they come from!)

That's why when health-care professionals make recommendations about what to eat and why, we're looking at all of the many factors that contribute to benefits and risks and making calculated recommendations by weighing when, what, how, and why an intervention may be right for you. It's my clinical opinion that while many keto enthusiasts claim it's not "restrictive," I beg to differ:

Limiting dietary carbohydrates is a form of restriction that *doesn't work well for everyone*. Depending on an individual's genetic makeup and normal activity level, a too-low-carbohydrate diet can have a negative impact on everything from energy levels to hormones. And often, the more you tell yourself you "can't have" something, the more you start to think about how much you're missing it, right? Plus, while the diet's not "low calorie," in theory, it's been mostly studied as such: Paoli and colleagues published a trial in *Nutrients* (2013) that was initiated with a significantly reduced-calorie ketogenic diet (<1,000 kilocalories per day), meaning that ketosis is initiated not only from the parameters of the diet, but also from what's known as a partial "starvation state" that also induces ketosis. Immediate and initial weight-loss results are therefore confounded by the facts that (a) subjects are taking in a lot less than they were before the trial, and (b) ketosis plays a role in increasing appetite-suppressing hormones. Sounds *awesome*, except that staying hydrated, sleeping, and exercising regularly (your biology sh*t starters!) are going to be compromised, and those too are responsible for appetite regulation (*best not to annoy them—they're feisty when they have low blood sugar!!*).

Here's the other thing: I'd encourage you to have a look at what's going on under the hashtag #keto via social media—there are beverages loaded with heavy cream, cheeseburgers without buns, and lots of processed meat with a side of lard. So while it may be possible to consume foods that are both in compliance with the diet and nutritious, the messaging around keto (and what makes it attractive to many, especially younger keto dabblers) is that you can basically eat tons of fast food and never have to choke down a vegetable again. I have some serious concerns about this, not the least of which is an eating pattern that is stringent enough to stunt growth and impact bones, skin, hair, nails, and teeth—which isn't going to be good for anyone (especially since keto can give you some aggressive halitosis already!).

Any eating plan that doesn't encourage higher quantities of vegetables and generally places caveats on real, whole foods limits the intake of fiber and micronutrients and, in addition to all of the many health risks, automatically becomes more expensive. While there are ways to cut back from a financial standpoint when going keto, you'd need to rely on daily supplements to meet micronutrient needs—which requires a pretty solid degree of financial security (*sounds a lot like a high barrier to entry, right?!*) and *disposable income*—a luxury not everyone enjoys. It's also not an eating plan that is holistically cognizant of how long-term reliance on diets *predominantly* consisting of *animal fat* affects our planet for the health of our family, friends, and future generations.

The bottom line is this: Diets such as keto or modified Atkins isolate specific nutrients from the context of our everyday lives (and limit you from the freedom of eating real, nutrient-dense foods in any given situation, no matter where you are in the world). They are shame-triggering recipes for failure, more fear, and more feelings of ineptitude and self-doubt. So, instead: What if we just skipped all of that and (a) ate some more vegetables and (b) moved our tushies just a few more times per day/week/month? Sounds a bit more fun, doesn't it, Sally?

Eating for the Long Haul

I feel strongly about the fact that a key measure of success with any diet plan is sticking with the general tenets of the diet for *life*—a diet that is too restrictive to maintain long-term can lead to weight-cycling—a cycle in which you gain a lot of weight when you're off the diet and lose a lot of weight when you're on the diet. Weight-cycling can lead to impaired glucose tolerance, chronic inflammation, and increased risk of cardiovascular disease, not to mention making weight loss *more difficult* each time you're back on the diet!

In order to keep that weight off, here are the things I'd like you to think about moving forward to keep your weight *and* biomarkers in a place that you and your physician feel is right, healthful, and empowering for you.

More Is More When It Comes to Veggies (and Fruit)

Adding more of these foods to your day, regardless of "net carbs," will be beneficial in reducing your long-term risk of chronic disease, will keep you satisfied (thanks to the fiber), and will aid in the management of GI-related side effects that you may (or may not—but I still have to say it!) have encountered during your time on any carb-restricted plan.

Consider the Type of Fat You're Eating

If you're at risk for diabetes, you're likely at risk for heart disease. That's why it's important to think about filling up on protein sources that contain good-for-you monounsaturated and polyunsaturated fats, which have been linked to reducing your risk of heart disease long-term. Since I'm not privy to your daily diet, it may be that you're doing this already. But just in case your meals *are* more heavily reliant on some keto staples, like bacon, butter, cheese, cream, and fatty cuts of meat and poultry—I'd encourage you to choose more fish and seafood, eggs, plant-based oils, nuts, seeds, beans, legumes, and avocado to make sure you're loading up on more balanced, nutrient-dense options that have been linked to improving cardiovascular function and blood sugar levels.

Incorporate Physical Activity into Your Repertoire

Blood sugar benefits, heart health, and overall weight management are achieved and maintained *mostly* through diet. But don't forget: calories in, calories out—burn more than you eat, you'll lose; burn less than you eat, you'll gain. That's why in addition to diet, it's important to add exercise for energy *balance* and to help burn any extra calories.

Bells, Whistles, and Why You (Might) Need Them

The Yerkes-Dodson law is a psychological theory developed in 1908 by, you guessed it—Yerkes and Dodson. These scientists proposed the idea that in order to achieve "optimal performance," we need a specific (not too low, not too high) level of cognitive "arousal," or motivation. The idea also supports a hormonal component, involving your glucocorticoids, which stimulate you *physically* to get your tush out of bed to do something you enjoy—thereby helping you to enjoy it *even more* (aka building momentum).

What does all of this have to do with your personal health and understanding which aspects of the whole "wellness world" may benefit you? Determining what specific elements of an activity or eating actually *motivate* you and help you to feel good about yourself physically and mentally—key factors in establishing good lifelong habits as they relate to taking care of your body.

Fun is crucial (science says so!). Yerkes and Dodson knew that in order to create behavioral change, we have to try things we enjoy that we'll be able to stick with, and be flexible in the process in order to accept new challenges that excite us. Think of it as the little bit *extra*—the little bit of frill attached to an action or activity that helps us enjoy doing it and actually making it a habit.

Frills can instigate just a teensy bit of motivation we need to experiment outside our comfort zones. Think of the recipes you'd like to try or the workout you'd love to make more regular. If you added on some frills—some more luxurious, elevated components to the experience— would you be more motivated to try it? For example: You spot a recipe with truffle oil and asparagus. You want to like vegetables, really, you do! But the only one you might consider liking just a little bit is asparagus. Here's where the frills, bells, and whistles come in. Does adding a delicious-tasting, decadent, and highly *frilly* oil make you want to eat those skinny green stalks?! (*If it does, then YAS!! Let's order it by the palette.*)

An even better way to think about this is the bells and whistles you may need (or detest!) to get you to work out.

Gyms aren't new (*the ancient Romans had those!*), but boutique fitness, like spin classes, for example, helps us escape, detach, and unplug for thirty minutes to an hour—something that's extremely desirable in a culture that craves just a teensy shred of "me time." Boutique gyms add a touch of luxury that feels indulgent, exclusive, and fun to something that can at times be monotonous and difficult (exercise). Let's explore cycling studios for a sec: fancy soap in the bathrooms, customer service at the front desk, and filtered water help turn a challenging workout into a delightful experience. What happens when you carve out a specific time slot in your day to have a treat-yourself type of experience with a group and you actually enjoy it? You go back again—and you keep going back. And it works when you stick with it.

If you're forking over a big chunk of money, suffering through those classes, rolling your eyes at the fragrant shower products, and resenting the heck out of everybody in a branded tank top, then you're not in an environment that's going to motivate you in a positive way. You're going to feel hugely relieved if you give yourself permission to find your own perfect balance, so define what those extras are for you, in the context of your life and the things you like to do, and go get 'em.

BELLS, WHISTLES, AND EXTRA FRILLS

If you need a lot of extras to get yourself to try something—food- or fitness-related—that is out of your comfort zone, or to make certain ho-hum activities feel more fun for you (Hey! Everyone needs a little schtick to get them to try something new!), try these suggestions:

- Check out new things one at a time, and in commitment stints that require some type of weekly or monthly financial renewal. To avoid eating the same things every day, for example, try meal delivery kits (Terra's Kitchen, Sunbasket, or Plated) that you subscribe to on a weekly basis and that provide all the fresh ingredients for you to try a new recipe. Or simply try doing a little planning as far as your schedule and shopping list go (see chapter 6) at the beginning of a week so you can try new recipes without the delivery kits.

- Apply a similar technique to your fitness routine. Maybe it would be worthwhile to try a different type of activity every time you exercise (e.g., spinning, tracking steps, or a digital fitness streaming service). Remember: Anything that (a) gets you to *move more* than what is status quo for you, and (b) excites you enough to commit to it is an overall benefit to your health and will help lead you to *other new things*. Don't be afraid to try 'em out!
- Think about other things that could make trying new recipes and attending boutique fitness classes appealing; for example, a new kitchen gadget or new workout clothes. Inspiration can come from small and unexpected places!

Shake up your snacks: I need a lot of schtick to get me to try new foods (recipes, restaurants, or ingredients), but I'm religious about my morning run.

Try scientifically backed, beneficial trends as follows:

- Ingredients that are trendy but are also *food* (not nutrients or supplements or powders). So long as you're eating them instead of drinking them, trendy ideas that meet the schtick sweet spot include premade or precut veggie/cauliflower rice and cauliflower pizza crust; other types of veggie rice; "zoodles" and other types of veggie noodles; legume-based pastas; and "bowls" that provide all of the ingredients but have *you* do the mixing in (e.g., Mann's Nourish Bowls).
- Meal delivery services that implement things mentioned above (e.g., Hungry Root).
- Desserts that use legumes as the flour base, like chickpea flour or black bean flour (e.g., black bean brownies or beet brownies) are great tools to help you introduce a new type of food or a new type of habit with flavors that are currently familiar.
- Snacks that use fruit (the type you chew instead of *drink*) but under a trendy moniker (e.g., fruit jerky).

Consider a monthly check-in re: your morning run whenever you feel like you're in a rut: Sign up for a race, think about hills versus sprints, or add a strength training component once a week. This can help you learn about new, running-adjacent activities that will help you be a better runner, won't overwhelm you with options or *schtick* overload, and can help you enjoy both running and a new activity even more.

Get a little "extra" with exercise: I need a lot of schtick to get me to try a new exercise class/routine/home workout, but my weeknight and weekend meals are pretty much predetermined (especially after chapter 4—Thanks, Jackie!)

- Consider opting in on group fitness of any kind via digital platforms, like ClassPass. This way, you'll pay for a standard subscription but will be able to try out more new things.
- Be wary of your own inclination to late-cancel on a class (a phenomenon that makes me personally *enraged*, but that's another story) for reasons that seem noble but are actually fear—and those roots run deep. You'll never know you hate it until you try it at least once—so think about the things that sound the most enjoyable to you and schedule them in small increments (once a week for one week; twice the next, etc.).
- Overwhelming yourself too much *with all of the frills* in relation to fitness can drain your resources—financially and physically—and give you a little burnout, so keep that in mind at the outset.

"Frills" and "Treats" Are Not Synonymous

The difference between having a little schtick involved as it relates to new habit formation and full-on *bribing yourself to do something* is the difference between what you're doing *during* the new thing you're trying and what happens once it's over. The difference is nuanced, but it's a crucial one. It defines the gap between *I'm going on a forty-minute walk/run so I can listen to this new podcast I love* and *I'm going on a long walk/run, and if I can get through it for forty minutes I'm treating myself to a carton of ice cream when I get home.* Why is this difference so crucial, you ask? Because if you train yourself to essentially receive a "reward" every time you do something that's challenging for you, there will come a time when you can't necessarily deliver on said reward—or at the very least, don't find it to be all that "healthy" for you, mentally, physically, or financially. In a reward model, you're only looking toward what you get at the *end*, instead of being motivated by the process itself. Really common examples of this in almost *all* of my clients include buying something new or indulging in something food-related that's been deemed "bad for you." It can seem innocuous at first, but how many times have we all said that, heard that, or seen it even in cultural examples?! "I just worked out so hard—I'm going to go and treat myself to a donut." Or, "I just ran a marathon in under four hours, so I'm buying myself a new car." These are great examples of ways that we can make ourselves feel good in a given moment. But can you afford to keep running races if every time you're going to run another one, your end goal is to buy an item that costs you more than what you make in a year? And are you really motivated to get up and run every single day to train for said race if all you get out of any given Wednesday morning five-miler is a stupid subway ride to the office and *not a damn* ~~Tesla~~ *Ford Focus*?! I think not.

I may sound like a broken record, but it's always worth repeating: *Even if you can sustain a new habit by consistently rewarding yourself at the end, there has to be SOMETHING rewarding about the process to make it worth sticking with long-term.* Plus, you've already tried this, remember?! You've done every diet and restricted all of the foods, and here we are! So that's why it's so key to know the difference between all of those frills to help you spring into action, and rewarding yourself with a treat for doing something you've deemed an obligation. Social media can have this wonky way of making us disassociate from what we actually like and feel as though we *should* like different things in order to reap a ~~bikini body~~ "reward." (To all of that noise, we say #byefelicia, and consciously *unfollow*.)

4

There's *Way Too Much* on My Plate Right Now to Think About Any Kind of "Self-Care"

After this chapter, you will...

- have a framework for maintaining your state of health—no matter what;
- manage your eating habits regardless of your schedule and time constraints; and
- take control of any relationships that have caused you to have some less-than-health-promoting feelings about food.

Strategies for Self-Care: A Beginner's Guide

Taking care of your health is a spectrum, and where you are on that spectrum at any given point in time is not stagnant—it will change with life stage, and it will *change daily*. There are always going to be days when you feel like you can barely brush your teeth, days when getting out of bed seems honestly impossible, and days when you feel like you could climb Everest (or at least get to Base Camp).

It's not up to me or anyone else to determine the degree to which you practice personal health, nor is it up to me or anyone else to judge how you're doing it today. But what I can (and will!) do is tell you to stop judging yourself, and I'm doing it by reminding you that (a) however much or however little you're doing to take care of yourself today does not determine what you'll do tomorrow, and (b) adapting to change is hard, but it's not impossible—especially when you remember that there's no point in trying to fit old habits into a new life stage.

So, let's embrace the change by strategizing how you can be a better, more adaptable caretaker for yourself—and be better equipped at taking care of other people and other things that need your help.

(Reminder: Everyone needs a little help sometimes.)

Self-care starts with prioritizing you as numero uno, making *your* well-being a priority. That involves developing clearly defined personal health goals that will inform the food and exercise choices you make. There's no balancing of energies, healing crystals, and prescribing yoga based on your astrological sign (unless you're into those, in which case, *you must be a mutable sign—me too!*).

Self-care is different for everyone, and it's as simple as a change in mind-set: If you're prioritizing your own health (mental, physical, and emotional), then you need boundaries to protect your plans. Let's begin with a little recap of the general basics.

In chapter 2 we discussed three factors that play significant roles in appetite regulation and play a more indirect role in how "in control" you feel over what you eat (that is, are you making a decision to eat that cookie, or do you feel like that cookie just owned you?!). These factors are:

1. sleep;
2. physical activity; and
3. hydration status.

Next, we covered the Right-Now Rules—the structure and framework you need to stick with any new change to your meals and snacks:

1. Eat breakfast every day (and make it bigger).
2. Don't skip meals or snacks (and make them satisfying).
3. Stay accountable (use tools that make it easier to eat better).

Cognitive Reframing

Regardless of whether you've already mastered the three Right-Now Rules or you're avoiding making any routine-changing health choices, now is the time to do a little cognitive restructuring. Reframing is an adaptive tool used in cognitive behavioral therapy (CBT) that helps to reinforce positivity (or for our purposes, stick to the basics of personal health and self-prioritization) when the going gets *hard* or your life circumstances change. What is CBT? Cognitive behavioral therapy is a psychotherapy technique that will help you identify and challenge strongly held beliefs and thinking patterns that are inaccurate or false, called *cognitive distortions*. Here's an example of what psychologists would call a *cognitive distortion*: "I can exercise only at the gym, and only if I can spin for forty-five minutes every single day like I did before I had my four kids!" You may be wondering, *What's distorted about that?* Well, my friends, listen up! Your circumstances have changed, but you want your exercise routine to stay the same—and that isn't working for you. (In fact, it's making you believe in a specific type of cognitive distortion called all-or-nothing thinking!) You believe regular exercise is impossible because your old routine won't fit into your current life stage or adapt seamlessly into your everyday lifestyle.

From a nutritional standpoint, we're going to cognitively restructure your thinking to maximize the two main areas of behavior change that help *all other habits* to gel. No matter what the circumstance, you prioritize these two things for yourself in whatever way possible (Spoiler: You *know* these already!):

1. Make *more* of your meals produce-based (aka more veggies and fruit; aim for at least half of your plate to be produce).
2. Move your tushy *more often* than you are right now (not necessarily barre, spin, marathon training; whatever you can do right now to just move—*do that!*).

Let's say a big part of your current self-care routine is tied to reading a book, newspaper, or magazine for as many minutes as you can possibly spare in any particular day, no matter the setting. How would you modify this self-care routine if you wanted to optimize it from the standpoint of making the two behavioral changes listed above?

Well, if this isn't your lucky day, I don't know what is—because the solution to your problem is right in your phone! Thanks to the digital world and earbuds, you're able to walk and listen to an audiobook or anything else you'd like. In fact, if you're listening to this book right now—well, kudos to you! Let's go for a walk together!

While I know I sound a bit like a cheese ball (or stick/cube/slice...), restructuring is key to establishing priorities, protecting boundaries, and doing so in a way that feels right for you. It requires you to look at your current lifestyle to make you aware of what you already do, and seek opportunities for modifying those things based on what you like—all in the framework of your daily habits and based on where you're at right now. Sometimes, that requires a little multitasking, and other times it means shutting down the blinds and going back to bed.

(Because, #balance, you know?!)

How exactly are you going to prioritize personal health when you have absolutely zero clue where to start? I'm glad you asked!

Step 1: Prioritize Personal Health by Assessing Your Daily/Weekly/Monthly Routine

Depending on where you are on this self-care spectrum, improving your personal health is your top priority (I mean, you wouldn't be reading this book if it weren't, right?!).

Whether you're just starting out with a new change or consider yourself a master of all things "personal health," beginning with these two weight loss–focused, health-promoting habits helps you come back to the basics of *energy balance*. In order to achieve weight loss, you have to actually use up more energy, or calories, than you've taken in to achieve a *negative energy balance*.

Remember: You bring yourself to the next "phase" of weight loss, maintenance, or better health with (a) more produce or (b) more movement.

Let's say you'd like to make more nutritious food choices, but you've been struggling because your current job requires dining out at lunches every week, at least four times per week. Your first step can be to decide a realistic number of times per week, number of eating occasions, or number of meals that you're committed to making more veg-heavy and develop a schedule based on your current routine that helps you put it into action. For example:

- You decide to add more veggies at lunch three out of the four days per week.
- You check your calendar to see where you're due to eat lunch, or suggest to your lunchmates where you'd like to go.

- You add a veggie-based salad, soup, side, or sauté that you'll include at each lunch. If that sounds too hard, scale back: Make it once per week, or decide not to do that at your lunch meal entirely (and make your goal to add more to your dinner instead, or fruit to your morning meal/vegetable to your omelet). If that sounds too simple, decide that you're going to add more produce at all meals this week, and make every meal heavy on the veg or fruit. (*If you are able to plan that far in advance, you're definitely an evolved human. I applaud you!*)

Modifications can be achieved over time by practicing what you're not sure you're capable of quite yet in smaller, more bite-size forms. (*Practice = confidence; confidence = habits and all, right?!*)

Next, we'll move on to managing this strategy and keeping up the momentum.

Other ways you can make current routines more movement-friendly:

1. Take one-on-one meetings out of the office while walking.
2. Take one-on-one meetings *in the office* while walking (real talk: I do this "indoor walk" with a coworker at least once per week; suspend all judgment till you try it, please!).
3. Building on 1 and 2 above, use networking time for "get-moving time." Consider how you might spend time with a coworker or a friend, going to a workout class or going on a walk or a run or a bike ride—doesn't matter, whatever gets you moving more, do *that*.
4. Pick up lunch from a location that's farther away than your usual (especially if "usual" = cafeteria down the hall).
5. If possible, walk to your workout class, sports practice, meeting in a different part of town, haircut, cobbler...you name it! Your new mantra: *"Walk early, walk often."*

Step 2: Set Boundaries That Will Help You Stick with a Schedule

Setting boundaries that help you stay in control of your own time and actions is the only way to stick to any new habit for the long-term, especially in the beginning when you're looking to try on a new change. No one else can do this part of *self-care* for you.

New routines require establishing habits that will ensure their success (meaning you can stick with them over time). That's why we're going to focus on goals in the realms of nutrient-dense eating and physical activity. If we were in my office together right now, I'd tell you this: On the spectrum of self-care and putting a new change into practice, *everyone* can focus on forming one new health habit at a time; *no one* can focus on *more than three* at a time, and all changes need a solid month to become a *habit* (we'll go through this step-by-step, which will help you feel less overwhelmed by the idea of a *whole month*).

Step 3: Identify Your Boundary Bullies (BBs)

Boundary bullies include stress, people, activities, and events that do their best to compromise your food and exercise choices. They can also come in the form of people, events, activities, and circumstances that make *you* feel required to put in a great amount of emotional or physical *energy* that is above and beyond the demands of your current existence (family, friends, job, general responsibilities of being a human being in the world, etc.).

In order for you to prioritize self-care through your established boundaries, it's important to identify your boundary bullies and specifically how and when they affect you. Ask yourself these questions:

1. **Where are my boundary bullies hiding?!** Start with a little assessment of your calendar—where are you physically at any hour, every day of the week? Finding your bullies is less difficult when you look at or think through your daily schedule, and add in the places where you spend most of your time—consciously or unconsciously. Take a moment to consider places you go in a given day that you could easily forget, simply because they're deeply ingrained in your routine. Are your boundary bullies secretly hiding at work? Are they in certain places or with certain people around the office? Are they at home? Are they in a club or sports league you belong to, or seemingly always at your a.m. coffee stop? (*Hello again, Tabitha!*)

2. **Who or what are they?** Once you've thought about *where* your food and exercise choices are usually compromised, it's easier to recognize *who* or *what* the BBs actually are. Make a list of which people and activities seem to be in the mix when you stray from your exercise and eating goals.

3. **Why are you getting bullied?** Once you know who and what these energy-zapping, progress-stunting vampires are and when and where they are most likely to strike, it will be a whole lot easier to figure out some defensive moves. Here are a few examples: Decide before your evening exercise class that you're going to say no to your friend's invitation to go out for a snack afterward. Adjust your work schedule at the office so if at all possible, you don't end up eating takeout at your desk. If you're with other parents, establish a plan with other moms to swap babysitting or playdate times, and if that doesn't work out, think of ways you can incorporate your exercise into your children's activities or during naptimes.

Doing this makes it easier to figure out the other things that fill up that energy tank instead of making you feel dread or depletion—and that's what we'll do next.

Step 4: Allow Your Schedule to Honor Your Boundaries

Remember when we talked about those totally real things that are basic biology and affect our ability to "stick with" a change or accept a new challenge? (Hint: We also called them your willpower sh*t starters):

- Dehydration
- Lack of sleep
- Changes in physical activity

Boundary bullies often manifest themselves by rabble-rousing behind the scenes and affecting any and all of these three appetite deregulators. For example: Your coworkers convince you to go get drinks after work instead of taking tonight off as you'd originally planned so that you can work out tomorrow morning. Now you're dehydrated from too many drinks and exhausted because you stayed out 'til 2 a.m. (wild!), and you skipped your workout because of all of that. End result? You feel a little bit like you're entering a shame spiral and you're also feeling physically *ravenous*.

To stave off these sneaky saboteurs: Entering your plan to leave work at a reasonable time, your plan to walk home from work, and the previously scheduled workout that's planned for 7 a.m. tomorrow is the first step to making your schedule meet your needs—and serve as border protection for your boundaries.

#protip

You're Numero Uno, Remember?!

Keep in mind that it's important to be wary of *shoulds* (chapter 1), which can sneak in as boundary bullies when you least expect it. For example, "I should sign up for this five-pack deal on barre classes because (a) SALE!! and (b) ABS!" But you never make it to said barre class because you realized that actually, you *hate* barre classes with a *fiery passion*! The bottom line: Just as there is a difference between an ambush annoyance and a boundary bully, there may also be multiple *shoulds* that you've allowed into your inner monologue unknowingly.

Doing this makes it easier to figure out the other things that fill up that energy tank instead of dread or depletion—protecting you from those *shoulds* that set you back.

Step 5: Have a Personal Ulysses Contract

If you've read or even just heard of the renowned classic *The Odyssey*, you may be familiar with the protagonist, Ulysses—whose journey across the Aegean Sea from Troy to Ithaca involves all manner of drama and adventure. At one point along his route, he travels by the Island of the Sirens and receives the warning: "If anyone unwarily draws in too close and hears the singing of the Sirens, his wife and children will never welcome him home again."

Ulysses decides to take a number of steps in order to stop himself from falling victim to the Sirens. They're so powerful, after all, that you can't just *unhear them*. They're *Sirens*! They're *seductresses*!

So what does Ulysses do to protect himself against the power of the magical Sirens? He gets himself a strategy! He has his crew put beeswax in their ears, making their hearts and heads impenetrable to the sounds of the Sirens. He ties himself to the mast of his *own ship* and instructs his crew to row—under any and all circumstances—so that they can remain safe and avoid the peril of the Island of the Sirens, where sailors wind up shipwrecked skeletons . . . just because they found themselves entrapped by monsters disguised as *supermodels*.

(*There's a great joke to be made in there somewhere, I'm sure.*)

When Ulysses's ship passes the Island of the Sirens, he hears their seductive singing, and he fights the ties that bind him; he *begs* the crew to untie him and let him steer the ship to get closer to them. But he physically cannot do so—he was *prepared* for this, so he's tied up six ways from Sunday. The crew (bless 'em) is rowing harder than ever—Ulysses warned them about this moment, and now here they are, speeding past the Island of the Sirens despite the angst and vitriol spouting from their fearless leader, who is *physically attached* to the center of the ship.

At long last, they pass the danger zone—and the sounds of the Sirens are faint calls in the background, barely audible. The crew stops rowing, and everyone begins to just *calm the f*ck down*.

This story has served as a metaphor in psychology and is even used in health-care practice today. It's called—you guessed it—the Ulysses contract, and it is a tool for taking steps in advance of an event to prepare yourself and others around you who are willing to help when you no longer feel as though you're in control. When the time came to brush close to danger, Ulysses didn't have to do all the work by himself. He had a plan of action already in place, set up by his logical self *ahead of time*. It worked for him, and it'll work for you.

Under duress, modern-day men and women can become susceptible to the siren call of stale Cheez-Its from the cupboard, cold pizza left over in the conference room, or picked-over brownies calling to us from the kitchen island. *Eat me! Eat me! Eat me!*

No adult is above the sirens of stress-eating. Not your family, not your friends, not your significant other, not your coworkers or your boss, and certainly not all the people in the world who make you think that it's not really a thing. (It *is*.) I'm a victim of it, every RD ~~worth meeting~~ I know has fallen victim to it, and anyone who tells you they *haven't*? Well, frankly I wouldn't trust them if I were you. (*Kidding! But seriously, how did you think health-care professionals survived organic chemistry?! Sour gummy worms are the foundation on which my entire career has been built.*)

But how can you do so without remorse and feeling as though you *chose* to do so?

Stress-Eating: Three Things You Need to Know

- Stress-eating is normal; routinely feeling out of control when you eat is not. (Consult your physician if you're concerned.)
- Stress-eating doesn't have to be an everyday thing.
- Stress-eating can be combated with mindfulness, and a lot of the time it's mitigated with your accountability tools—assessing where you are on the FNSS scale—and evaluating your level of hunger, hydration, exhaustion, and mood can help you figure out whether what you really need is a snack, a glass of water, or a walk around your office building.

Step 6: Rule Out Biology Before Taking Action

Ultimately, my only hard rule for ensuring that these self-care strategies actually work is to make sure you stick to ruling out the physical reasons why you might be eating, aka your biological sh*t starters (One more time! For the cheap seats in the back): You're exhausted; you didn't exercise enough/exercised too much/changed your entire exercise routine/need to get up for a walk; or you're dehydrated.

So, start here:

- Have a 16-ounce glass of water.
- Go out for a coffee, tea, or some other caffeinated beverage (aim for about 100 mg, more or less, depending on how much sleep you're racking these days, or how caffeine-sensitive you are) and make sure it's unsweetened.

If you did get enough sleep for you last night (but are feeling desperate for a snack, despite the fact that you just ate), take a walk that's a minimum of fifteen minutes, preferably with a colleague who you can cajole into taking a break with you. Why? This is what research tells us is the most satisfying, emotionally recharging form of a break, which can help you assess if you do actually need more food, or if you just needed said walk and time to catch up with…you guessed it…Bob! From *accounting*! (Bob enjoys a sensible fifteen-minute stroll around the neighborhood, too, you know.)

Next, let's move on to the food-related biological reasons you might be uncharacteristically ravenous in any given stressful moment:

- You didn't eat breakfast (or you did, but it was basically a sad breakfast biscuit and black coffee, aka *not enough*!).
- You skipped a meal or skipped a satiety-boosting combo of foods at your last meal (see above re: your sad, fiberless breakfast biscuit and ~~semi-burnt~~ coffee).
- You opted out of all the tools listed in chapter 2 (*Come on, guys!*).

First, where are you on the satiety scale?

- If you're above a 4 (but below a 6 on the FNSS scale): You need a *snack*.
- If you're above 6: You need more of a nosh—how about a few of those chocolates (on page 106)?
- If you're anywhere below a 4: You need a *sneal*.

WTF Is a Sneal?

No, I'm not telling you to read a Dr. Seuss book. (But on that note, why not? Self-care takes many forms.) Actually, a sneal is a cross between a snack and a meal—it's about 250 to 300 calories, and it's the solution to your problems when you're kinda hungry, kinda anxious, but have skipped a meal or had a rather incomplete set of meals (missing one or both fiber and protein) that has led you to experience that whole "I'm full but I'm not satisfied" syndrome (and drew you to thinking about food in the first place); or, you skipped a meal (or self-restricted on your last few meals!) because you're waiting on your next big meal where you think you'll be eating "too much."

The problem with that strategy is that without a snack or a sneal at this moment, you're *primed* to stress-eat just about everything in your line of sight. (*Watch out, manila folders—you look like you could sub for sandwich bread.*)

Instead, have some snacks on hand that can, when necessary, be combined into sneal format. Sneals on hand at the office and at home will keep you in check until you can have a full, nutritious meal rather than trying to use the mythical "willpower" to just have a handful of crackers on loan from Diane. That's a waste of time, and a waste of calories you could spend on eating something more enjoyable, more nutritious, *and* more satisfying.

Try a Better Band-Aid: Understanding "Cravings"

Traditional diet culture loves the word *craving*. According to *Merriam-Webster*, a craving is "an intense, urgent, or abnormal desire or longing." First of all, OUCH, *Merriam*! "Abnormal?" *Really?* (We were burned by "superfood," and we've been burned *again*.)

Too often we lose sight of exactly where cravings come from—are they emotional (stress-induced; looking for the mood-boosting effects of chocolate or sugar; a way of saying, "Screw it!") or physical (an actual need to supply a missing or insufficient nutrient) or a combination of the two (in addition to the mood-boosting effects of chocolate, for example, it also supplies magnesium)?

Maybe you feel an urgent need to eat ice cream or you intensely desire something salty. Is that abnormal? Nope. Often, the more we restrict or exist in a constant state of *white-knuckling it*, the more our bodies biologically crave the nutrients we're missing. On top of that, if something hectic or unexpected happens, taking us away from our ability to use the Band-Aid compensatory strategies that temporarily meet our needs, we simply don't know what to eat and thus turn to the foods that are either readily available to us (Wheat Thins in the office) or highly comforting (cupcakes from the local bakery).

Real talk: As a clinician, it's my experience that in addition to all of the science, cravings come from the absence of something—not the need for an addition of something *else*. There are medical conditions and states of health that can lead you to feel like you want something you've never eaten before in your life, and very legitimate biological reasons why you feel as though you need to eat a particular flavor of something. When cravings are not biological, though, they're usually related to FNSS (full-but-not-*satisfied* syndrome).

When you're missing a macronutrient from a meal (protein, fat, or carbs in the form of fiber), you might find yourself grazing or staring at the fridge, waiting for the revelation of what you can eat that will magically make you feel "sated," even though you can barely breathe because you're super full. Haven't we all been there? This happens when we eat predominantly carbs *alone* (e.g., pasta with tomatoes or tomato sauce) or when we eat protein *alone* (steak, hold the potato!). That's why meals and snacks need to be at least 50 percent produce to maximize on fiber (and as part of your self-care plan, you're adding an increasing amount of these babies to meals and snacks, right?!), with some lean protein and some healthy fat. This *satiety trifecta* of nutrients helps us really get in touch with why we want to eat—because if you skip the carbs for a diet-related reason and missed out on a perfectly reasonable sweet potato at lunchtime, it's highly likely that eventually you'll want them in the form of cake.

Stress-Induced Procrastin-eating

Confession: I'm procrastin-eating hard-core as I write this chapter. In fact, I just went back for a few more of the trusty sour gummy worms!

Procrastin-eating is what happens when you're seriously putting off something you have to do, and you start to think about eating instead of just doing the damn thing. Examples of procrastin-eating instigators might include not wanting to work on your taxes, prepare an expense report, write an email, pay bills, or make a to-do list. Sound familiar?

Sometimes all you lose is a few minutes before you get back to the grind. But other times, if you're anything like me, you go a step further and lose an entire half day to procrastin-*cooking* (*that one doesn't work as well... but you know what I mean*).

So, can you avoid it? Of course you can! If you need to take a break, or delay starting on whatever it is you need to do but really don't want to do, there are many more things to try to occupy your time besides snacking.

Here's how to artfully procrastin-eat:

- Prepping versus eating: Use time during which you'd otherwise procrastin-eat to prepare for another meal (e.g., chop garlic, shuck corn, boil beets—to prep ahead for dinner. *Notice how all of those are vegetables? Not an accident.*).
- Take a walk to get yourself away from the food you're tempted to eat. This one is your proverbial meat and potatoes—eat your heart out.
- Split up a meal and build it into procrastin-eating: Save half of your sandwich at lunch and procrastin-eat the hell out of it while going through the remains of your email mountain (or avoiding that looming expense report.

Splash Mountain Syndrome (aka, I'm Too Stressed to Eat)

Motion aside, going to theme parks and partaking in (way-too-scary-for-me-but-maybe-fun-for-you!) rides like Splash Mountain fires hormones in our bodies that make us nervous, excited, and ultimately, exhilarated. On a biological scale, that looks like this: You anticipate an event that makes you feel all the feelings—nervous, excited, and ultimately…exhilarated. When your brain stimulates your glucocorticoids, it's tough to get a handle on your *real* appetite versus your triggered feelings of hunger and satiety.

Many people *do* feel like they're too stressed to eat at times, and that's a perfectly normal biologically driven response to stress. While some of us can "grin and bear it" and eat when we're not all that hungry, others find it completely impossible. What can help a stress-induced lack of appetite? I usually recommend one of two strategies for this, depending on who you are and what it is that's making you anxious. The first one works for people who like structure—you have a schedule that you like sticking with, and on top of what is causing your stress-induced lack of appetite, the feeling that you're messing up your own normal patterns and lifestyle is even more anxiety-provoking, which can lead to overeating during random moments of stress relief. The second strategy works for those who feel too stressed to eat all day at work, and then wind up overeating once they get home at night.

1. Break every meal you'd normally eat in half. Say, for example, that you normally have oatmeal with nuts, seeds, and fruit for breakfast. Start your day with the hot oats, sweeten 'em up with a little fruit, and move the nuts and seeds to somewhere around 10 a.m. (or whatever your one to two hours later looks like). If you're planning on having a sandwich for lunch, halve it. Same with dinner: Make a stir-fry and put half away in the fridge. Since stress can also instigate a range of tummy troubles, I'd go heavier on the protein for dinner part one, add as many veggies as you'll feel like you want to eat there, and then save the rest for later.

2. High-quality grazing can work as a strategy to keep you from overdoing it at night. The key to this technique is storing snacks (nutrient-dense things you know you like to eat in any frame of mind) in places where they're visual during daytime hours when you're feeling said anxiety. These snacks won't feel like a meal individually, but they can add up to one—meaning you're making a conscious choice to fuel yourself during the day (despite a lack of hunger) so you won't feel like a bottomless pit at dinnertime.

Some of you can eat only certain "safe" foods when you're super anxious or feeling upset, and that's completely legit, too. Here are some foods that most people tolerate really well when feeling *too stressed to eat*:

1. Tea or milk: Add low-fat or skim milk to the tea for a more filling beverage. One cup of soy, pea, or cow's milk provides 7 to 8 grams of protein, which will help you feel more satisfied when the anxiety or upset dissipates and you're ready to eat the actual cow.
2. Apples/applesauce: Eat apple slices whole or mix applesauce into oats and add a tablespoon of chia seeds; then let it sit overnight for a nutritious, satisfying snack or meal that won't upset your tummy.
3. Bananas: Bananas + yogurt + ice = smoothie. You can try adding nut butter or cottage cheese to boost the nutritional quality of your snack without overdoing it.

4. Eggs/egg whites: Eggs have a nutritionally perfect composition of high biological value protein, antioxidants, and healthy fat. Eat them with avocado on your toast.

5. Crackers/toast: Adding avocado, nut butter, or part-skim cheese can make a light meal of toast or crackers more balanced and help keep your energy up so you don't completely crash later on.

Decide When "Good" Is Better Than "Best"

When it comes to indulgences, a lot of people subscribe to the advice to keep them at arm's length: "Throw away the rest of the pizza so you don't have to see it after you've eaten one slice!" "Ruin your dessert after you take a few bites so you won't eat the rest!" and of course, "Do *not*, under any circumstances, keep treats in your house!" These suggestions *can* work, but only temporarily—they will, almost 100 percent of the time, come back to bite you in the tush. The idea is that if it's there and it's a trigger for you, you *will* inherently go back to it. But there's another part of this to consider, too, and that's the fact that taking the "stigma" out of these foods is something that can only happen the more you keep the idea of satiety top of mind. When you're operating out of FNSS, sure—certain foods *become triggers* (poor cereal or popcorn or chocolate-covered anything weren't born that way—sorry, guys!). At the same time, certain brands or types of foods don't have to be unilaterally maligned. For example, let's take my favorite condiment, peanut butter.

Peanut butter is the world's most perfect food as far as I'm concerned. There are memes all over social media like "peanut butter is the glue that holds my life together," and I couldn't agree more! A 2-tablespoon serving of PB is full of the satiety trifecta. Not all brands are the same, of course, but a good median nutritional value would consist of protein (8 g), fiber (4 g), and healthy fat (22 g). Each serving also contains approximately 200 calories, which in itself makes it a super-*filling* food—but the fact that those calories come from all three nutrients in ample amounts means it can keep you fuller *longer*. And when you add additional fiber from whatever you're eating with it (e.g., an apple, celery, bread, etc.), that staying power is amplified.

But when you're suffering from FNSS and operating on an *unsatisfied* stomach after noshing on countless stale "For Sharing" crackers, that's when you're primed to eat half the jar of peanut butter rather than a reasonable serving. Why? Because you didn't close the loop of the satiety "trifecta." Instead, you found carbs, but no good protein, fiber, or fat! It's no wonder the peanut butter jar (or baking supplies, or soufflé, or anything else that should find its way into your home at any given time or place) turns from regular food into "trigger food" in this situation; it's delicious and creamy, and the mouthfeel of high-fat foods is heavenly.

The best tip I can give you on how to reroute yourself when you're on your way to the bag of chips or leftover Halloween candy is to pause and think a little bit more about what you're actually in the mood to eat—and think of what you'd want to solve it. Do some strategic thinking on a full stomach and consider what foods you reach for when this type of hankering comes on. Then get creative about keeping nutritious snacks on hand that will help satisfy your usual cravings.

Sometimes there are items that feel (for whatever reason or none at all!) too easy to overeat, and you feel like it's completely impossible to resist the temptation to overeat them. So don't fall for it by deciding what's good enough to quell the "I really want chocolate" feeling with something that you like eating (let's say M&M's) but that isn't so unbelievably delicious to you as a Cadbury Crème Egg. Finding this distinction is a great strategy to determine whether or not you want to empower "screw it" as a decision. If you're satisfied by the M&M's, you're good to go. If you really just wanted a jumbo-size crème egg after thinking about the M&M's (or even trying a piece or two?), well then, screw it! Go for it and love every delicious bite.

Empower "Screw It!" to Be a Decision

Often we find ourselves feeling unsatisfied rather than sated by eating a stupid piece of fruit when what we actually wanted was dessert. We didn't get specific about the flavors we wanted, nor did we think through how we might be able to satisfy our craving in a way that has meaningful, realistic, and *filling* properties! The best tip I can give for how to reroute yourself when you're on your way to the bag of chips or leftover Halloween candy is to pause and think a little bit more about foods you're actually "craving." Be strategic when you're thinking on a full stomach and consider what foods you like to eat and what foods you reach for when the bingies start to come on. Then get creative about making meals and snacks that satisfy the flavor you love while adding in more nutritious options.

STRESS-EATING SWAPS

If You Stress-Eat Baked Goods: Keep Single-Serve Candies on Hand

Lollipops: 1 pop = 60 calories; 0 g saturated fat; 15 g sugar

Why they're legit: They take longer to eat! Keeping one of these handy to pop into your mouth might keep you from going nuts with the candy corn. Plus, since it takes a while to get to the center, you'll have more time to get in tune with your body's satiety cues postmeal.

York Peppermint Patties: 2 patties = 120 calories; 1.5 g saturated fat; 22 g sugar

Why they're legit: The chocolate-mint combo is like a special after-dinner treat. The dark chocolate plus mint filling makes these taste both satisfying and indulgent, without breaking the bank on calories or saturated fat.

Fun-Size Pretzel M&M's: 3 packs = 150 calories; 3 g saturated fat; 17 g sugar; 2 g protein; 1 g fiber

Why they're legit: Crunchy and super satisfying (you get three whole bags?!). If you're not a fan of this fluffier, lighter M&M, the peanut M&M's are okay too—they pack 5 g of protein in a full bag (240 calories) for when you're in the mood for something more satisfying.

Mini Snickers or **Fun-Size Snickers:** 4 mini or 2 fun-size = 170 calories; 3 g saturated fat; 18 g sugar; 3 g protein; 1 g fiber

Why they're legit: Snickers really are more satisfying, thanks to peanuts, which bring the protein up to 3 g/serving.

Hershey's Kisses: 7 to 9 Kisses = 150 calories; 6 g saturated fat; 17 g sugar.

Why they're legit: Simple and delicious! These are high-volume (200 calories in nine!), but they also require unwrapping—which slows you down as you snack, giving you more time to digest and feel satisfied.

If You Stress-Eat Burritos, You Should Keep Avocados/Salsa/Beans/Greek Yogurt/Bagged Salad Greens on Hand

Let's walk through what you like best about a burrito: You probably love the burrito's creamy, hearty, and spicy mix of flavors, as well as the guacamole on top. When you're in the mood for something healthy that has the flavor of a burrito, your best bet is to opt for the ingredients that make a burrito what it is: avocado, salsa, hot sauce, beans, part-skim shredded cheese, and maybe some extra tomatoes, plus a dollop of Greek yogurt—but instead of filling a flour tortilla with these items, add them to a bowl of salad greens. This way you're getting the same flavor that you're craving, but not the overloaded, food-coma-inducing combo of all these ingredients plus saturated fat, sodium, and refined carbs from rice and the tortilla. The idea here is that you're creating a lighter version of something you like—but it's still high in protein, low in saturated fat, and lower in sodium, and it maximizes the flavors you enjoy having.

If You Stress-Eat Pizza, You Should Keep Ingredients for DIY Pizza on Hand

Buy shredded part-skim cheese, low-sodium jarred tomato sauce, and 2% cottage cheese. For the crust, try any of these options in 100 percent whole-grain form: pita bread, English muffins, bagel thins, or sandwich thins.

Toss on any combo of frozen veggies or fresh-cooked veggie leftovers—these will help to fill you up. The idea behind this hack is that you're essentially making a veggie-heavy grilled cheese (extra delicious if you drizzle a little olive oil on here and "grill" the bread!), but nipping the desire to go with takeout.

If You Stress-Eat Fries, You Should Keep Frozen Baked Alternatives on Hand

Green Giant, Alexia, Trader Joe's, and Whole Foods 365 brand oven-baked versions aren't totally deep-fried but still retain the "fry" texture, shape, and quality. Look online for recipes to create your own version of baked vegetable fries. These are a great way for you (and your kids) to try new veggies and flavor combos, and you can serve these as a side dish no matter where your level of stress sits!

5

I Can't Lose Weight Because of My Genetics/Family/ Relationship/Job

This chapter will teach you...

- how to shut down the inner food pushers that make you feel powerless against the munchies;
- how to enjoy foods you love without feeling out of control; and
- how your habits can help you make decisions about what you eat.

People, Proximity, and Deciding What to Eat

One thing that always struck me in clinical practice and private counseling was how the health status of other family members played a tremendous role in a willingness to change health habits. Some days it truly seemed that *every client* felt their health and eating habits were influenced in some way by family (especially spouses), friends, or colleagues. It was certainly a less frequent occurrence on such days to sit down and talk to a client about making food and health decisions that would *affect only them*. That's why we've got to cover some scenarios that are common for all of us, and are (mostly) unavoidable, are (often) stressful, and (always) involve the influence of people other than you. (Because it's not all about you, Ethel! The foods you eat aren't always the ones you'd choose if you were left to your own devices!)

Family Medical History

Fact of life: Your medical history is not necessarily your own—your family may have a history of type 2 diabetes, or perhaps you come from the esteemed lineage of the gastrointestinally challenged. But just because everyone in your family developed insulin-resistance (aka prediabetes) does not 100 percent seal your fate! You *do* have some food-related influence over your genes in these areas:

- Diabetes
- Heart disease
- Lifestyle-related cancers
- Chronic kidney disease/fatty liver disease
- Alzheimer's disease and cognitive decline
- Overweight/obesity
- Hypothyroidism
- Neuromuscular disease/autoimmune disease
- Depression/mood disorders

But there is an important thing to remember here, too: Your genes are out of your control (sorry about that!), but you *can* change your habits as a result of knowing a thing or two about your DNA. This is not to say that changing your habits guarantees you won't develop diabetes, cancer, or the high blood pressure that runs in your family. But *not* taking some steps to protect yourself could increase your risk of developing health issues later on! Beyond that fact: The greatest gap in knowing that you'd like to make a change and actually putting that change into action is a little *F* word called *fear*. And in my experience, anyone who is afraid to make changes as they relate to their health is often (even if it's just a little bit!) stuck in the info jungle: It feels hard because what you've heard in the past really seems that way! But relax, you're here now, my friends! Understanding your past medical or family's medical history can help you make easy and delicious choices that serve your present and your future.

#protip

Accountability

Here's an example of a dynamic that would cross my path *at least* once a week during clinical practice: A couple, one of whom had been diagnosed with a heart-disease-related risk factor, came (sometimes, directly!) from the cardiologist's office to see me. In most cases (and given census stats on men, women, and heart disease), the client would be the husband, accompanied by his wife, who was always there to "take notes" or "just listen." These clients were *always* the most likely to stick with any specific plan, eating style, or other medical nutrition therapy I'd recommend—and I would see some amazing results in a shorter period of time than in the clients flying solo. Accountability is key to making any behavioral change, but it also shows how a patient's accountability to the person or people closest to him or her stimulates changes in both parties.

Your Metabolic Rate

After the age of thirty, your muscle mass declines by about 5 percent per decade. But that 5 percent pertains to *one biological factor* that plays a role in metabolic rate. The other factors of your basal metabolic rate—thermic effect of food, physical activity energy expenditure, and resting energy expenditure—can be manipulated by increasing how much you burn through activity, and the offset of lean body mass (aka building muscle).

It's actually quite glorious—because, frankly, there's so much in the world that we *can't* control, but the fact that we have some agency in increasing our own metabolism even slightly, or burning just 100 *more calories* in a day, is one pretty awesome thing to put into the category of "stuff over which we have control."

Since we're all starting from a different place: Use these ideas as a general metric from which you can build upon or scale back, but notice that each, though they're examples, provides a specific time frame with a specific action:

- Schedule in a strength training session every Wednesday for thirty minutes (10 prework, 10 at lunch, 10 while you're preheating the oven for dinner tonight).
- Walking five days a week? Add ten minutes to your routine on three of those days.
- Five-day-a-week runners: Go for your usual run, but increase the intensity with two hills, two minutes each on Mondays and Fridays.
- Twenty squats during each commercial break during Monday night #BachelorNation. (*Time flies when you're squatting with Chris Harrison!*)

See what we're doing here? The idea is that you're being specific about your schedule to achieve a more specific goal. Change the numbers, times, dates—but go back to your 80:20 ratio—this should feel difficult enough based on where you're at to excite you by the challenge, but not so out of your wheelhouse that you're overwhelmed by the idea of it.

Your Personal Food History

Your current food preferences are most likely a product of lifelong or long-term eating habits of a specific range of foods that you enjoy and are comfortable eating. Adding new and possibly healthier foods to your diet can take some dedication and perseverance. Perhaps as a kid you did not have much exposure to, say, *fennel*, so you've decided you don't like it. Or maybe there are certain foods that you pass on because you had a bad encounter. It's important to check in with yourself and those foods, though, because you will likely surprise yourself. For me personally, that was cucumbers. I had hated them my whole life. But then one day I tried eating some cucumber again and decided that it's really quite innocuous! *Who knew?!* The benefits of stepping outside your comfort zone are many, but to name two important ones: It will help you form a habit of trying different things, and it will reinforce the lesson that the rules of the past don't have to dictate the future.

Preferences aren't stagnant—they often evolve over time. So check in with yourself every now and then and give that food you thought you didn't like a retry—maybe *more than once or twice*. You might find that you actually enjoy it! Experiment with different cooking methods and oils, spices, even raw versus cooked to see if that changes your opinion of the food. You'll be fostering a sense of open-mindedness when it comes to how and what you eat.

Food preferences are normally based on taste likes or dislikes, but food associations, which we'll cover next, are a result of emotions and feelings being connected to food.

What's a Food Association?

Food associations evoke feelings—positive, negative, or a mixture of both. Lifelong food associations, positive and negative, are often formed in early childhood. Food associations can also be triggered by experiences and events in adulthood.

A negative food association that's very base-level and clear would result from eating a food and then becoming ill as a result of a foodborne illness or the food just not agreeing with you for some reason (FYI, mine's Raisinets—showing me a chocolate-covered dried grape reminds me of a stomach flu I had during elementary school after I downed those ~~rabbit-droppings~~ candies while watching the movie *Hook*. This whole thing went down *decades* ago, and yet when someone even utters the word *Raisinet*, my throat closes up and I get that *Am I going to be sick?!* feeling at the bottom of my sternum).

Food associations can actually be media-created, too. Being bombarded by information regarding what's "good for you" versus what's "bad for you" and what "*superfoods* you *should be eating right now*" can make you feel that certain foods *must* be a part of your diet, while other foods *must* be eliminated completely. These fads can permeate an entire generation's attitude toward certain foods—millions of people avoiding bread because "carbs make you fat"; eating celery because it "burns more calories than it contains"; eating only fat-free products that are basically salty air (and therefore you eat a zillion more of them than you would otherwise!).

Positive food associations play a role in your eating habits, too, and those are the ones to keep at the forefront of your inner monologue. Sharing food, or "breaking bread," with friends and family can be one of life's most enjoyable experiences. An example of how food companies have capitalized on one positive food association: birthday cake! Most people connect eating birthday cake with happy, carefree times. So now there are birthday-cake-flavored protein bars, ice cream, cookies, peanut butter, milkshakes, popcorn—there are even birthday-cake-flavored condoms these days!

Your negative food associations may play a small role in your everyday life, or they may be driving you to avoid entire meals, eliminate certain foods, or adhere to stringent rules—without you necessarily realizing you're doing it. Examine your negative food associations and acknowledge their existence. Are you wondering why you hate Easter brunch *so damn much* or why you consider pancakes the most dreadful food in the world? Dig deep: Could there be a reason *why* you feel like this? Did some sh*t *seriously hit the fan* at Easter brunch somewhere around sixth grade? Did your mom eat pancakes *only* when she was at an emotional rock bottom? There's nothing you can do about the fact that these things happened, but acknowledging the role they play in your food choices *today* can help you to manage them and cultivate a greater level of safety in discussing them.

When it comes to both food preferences and food associations, the best way to manage these factors right now, in present-day life, is to consider customization to meet your specific needs in any given scenario. Customization is about to become your best friend—and it's much easier than it sounds.

An example I hear frequently (mostly from parents!) sounds like this:

Everyone under my roof eats different things, and we can't make a decision on dinner. Any ideas?

Customizing a meal does *not* mean turning your kitchen into a restaurant at mealtimes; it's about preparing meals with nutritious ingredients that can be consumed in varying quantities depending on taste. Start with the bases:

Rice, potatoes, and pasta are three examples of foods that can, in fact, be prepared nutritiously. Here's how:

Rice: Luckily for you (and *every single parent under the sun*), there is a kind of renaissance happening with the "ricing" of vegetables. Cauliflower, kohlrabies, parsnips, turnips, white carrots, and even jicama are all examples of foods that are (a) vegetables and (b) white (like rice). Tons of food companies, chain supermarkets, and even restaurants are producing riced versions of these foods, meaning that you don't have to spend hours trying to make cauliflower rice with a head of this cruciferous vegetable and a cheese grater (one client of mine tried this once—and all he got was a hot mess in the kitchen and two hours of his life missing forever).

You can make the switch completely by simply nuking up some cauliflower rice or other vegetable rice and seasoning to your heart's desire, or you can introduce this new flavor gradually in ⅓-cup increments. Add ⅓ cup of veggie rice to each ⅔ cup of traditional rice, and increase the proportion from there until it's 100 percent veggie rice.

Pasta: A common question that I received from clients when I worked in private practice and continue to receive in my current position at GH is "How can I eat pasta and still lose weight?" Thanks to some seriously smart food scientists, legume-based pastas are the wonderful answer to said question. Pulse crops (e.g., beans, lentils, chickpeas, and peas) can be made into flour used to make pasta, bread, and other baked goods. The reason pulse flours are nutritionally optimal as compared to traditional wheat flour is that they contain extra fiber and plant-based protein—up to 20 grams of each per every 2 ounces.

Twenty grams of protein is about the size of a Mac computer mouse of beef, chicken, or fish. Combine legume-based pastas with veggies, sauce, and additional protein if you're aiming for a meal that is not only filling but also nutrient-dense. Pulse-flour pastas are also a good way to introduce a slightly different flavor experience to your family.

Root veggies: Mashed versions of root veggies such as cooked or baked carrots, parsnips, turnips, taros, or any combination are nutritious and delicious. With a little extra mashing, basically any other vegetable can be incorporated into the dish, too.

Vegetable pasta bar or loaded baked potato bar: With the pasta and potatoes as the blank canvases, this is all about the toppings and little effort from you. Think roasted and fresh veggies, cheeses, tomatoes/tomato sauce, pulses (e.g., beans, chickpeas, lentils), olive oil, spices, herbs, onion, Greek yogurt—use your imagination.

Snacks: The key to life is compromise, am I right? So when it comes to snacks, buying packaged versions of things that often feel like a treat, or combining part deliciousness and part nutritious deliciousness is your go-to hack. Again, a little bit of prep goes a long way. For example: Fruit skewers can be a fun way to get your kids excited about fruit for a snack because they're much like ice pops (especially when you freeze them). Good fruits to slide on the skewers include berries; tropical fruits like papaya, mango, and pineapple; watermelon; and clementine slices. Before serving, sprinkle with coconut flakes or white chia seeds to make them just a bit more filling and attractive.

Other healthy snack ideas include:

- Veggie- or fruit-based "sandwiches": sweet potato plus nut butter; banana slices plus nut butter.
- Fruit and veggie chips: Try Bare Snacks, Rhythm Superfoods, or Terra.
- Veggie-based muffins: Garden Lites and Soozy's are two great brands of veggie-filled baked goods that can be stored in the freezer and prepared as a snack for your kids (and all of their friends) in under one minute in the microwave.
- Smoothies and smoothie bowls: Blending fruit with milk for a drinkable snack makes for a fun foray into the world of fruit for kids. Use any type of fruit, or a combination of two or three types, add milk, and blend. You can also make a heartier snack by adding nuts (if tolerated), fresh fruit, coconut, and chocolate to a smoothie bowl. Top with a "fairy dust" blend of flaxseeds and chia seeds. You can even call it superpower dust! Because anything that gets your kids to eat more produce is *super powerful* in itself!
- "Pizza": The good news is that pizza is a vehicle for vegetables. Introducing a new veggie on top of a snack pizza is a great way to get your little ones to give it a try. Melt some cheese on whole-grain bread, pita, or crackers as your base. Customize the toppings based on your kids' level of interest in trying some new, nutritious things.

- Cereal: Cereal serves as a go-to snack for many, and nutritious toppings such as seeds, nuts, and shredded or flaked coconut are natural additions, along with fruit (strawberries, raspberries, peaches, and pineapple are all delicious in cereal).

Why am I the only person eating the brussels sprouts and there's a fight over the mac 'n cheese?

Truth: A strong-tasting vegetable is in a lonely battle with items traditionally considered "comfort food" on the table. Give the following ideas a try if you want to make vegetables more accessible and appealing to the whole clan.

Make Vegetable Soup

Hot or cold soup is an ultrasimple way to get the whole family to eat more veggies. Use your favorite recipes and double up on the nonstarchy stuff (e.g., broccoli, cauliflower, celery, carrots, tomatoes, fennel, mushrooms, spinach) or try out a cold vegetable soup like gazpacho, which can be super satisfying once the hot weather hits.

Add Vegetables to Pasta Sauce

Sauté diced eggplant or eggplant slices (not an eggplant lover? Try this with mushrooms, spinach, or zucchini!) with tomatoes, garlic, and a dash of olive oil until tender. You can use this mix as a pasta sauce or add it to your favorite jarred low-sodium tomato sauce as a way of slipping extra veggies into *any* pasta dish! It's a great way to introduce kids (even *adult* kids) to new veggies. Plus, the added fiber from the vegetables bulks up your meal, so you'll feel more satisfied.

Use Vegetable Spreads

PB&J is a time-honored classic (and one of my personal favorites!). But did you know that all kinds of vegetables, sometimes combined with yogurt rather than mayo or cream cheese, and with just the right seasonings, make a wonderful sandwich (or bagel, or pita, or muffin thin) spread? Check out the recipes available online for ideas!

Turn Vegetables into Dippers or Chips

Who says veggies can't also be a vehicle for your favorite spreads and dips? Sliced cucumbers, radishes, jicama, and asparagus spears are great dipped into guacamole or hummus—especially the red pepper and garlic-flavored versions—or dip them into your favorite Greek yogurt–based dip for some extra protein. Another trick to try: Make kale chips or sweet-potato fries, which you can whip up in under twenty minutes!

Try Vegetables as Toppings

Shaved, roasted brussels sprouts or kale on stir-fries and sautés make for an extra veggie-based hit of flavor. But don't stop there—we love adding crunchy veggies to whole-grain crackers with cheese for a snack, doubling up on veggies as pizza toppings, or sprinkling fruit on overnight oatmeal and yogurt parfaits. Another tip: Don't be afraid to top savory meals with the sweetness from fruit (and vice versa!). Papaya or mango is great in spicy stir-fries, while adding steamed tomatoes, spinach, or kale to (traditionally sweet) hot cereal breakfasts can be a fun take on an old staple. (Insider tip: We love these topped with a poached egg, too!)

Try a Little "Mash"

As noted above under "Root veggies," vegetables can be mashed into creations that rival any regular mashed-potato dish for flavor and nutrition!

Layer Vegetables on Sandwiches

Sprouts and carrots and tomatoes—oh my! Load up any sub or sandwich with your favorites for extra flavor (and obviously, high-fiber fillers that will help you stay full and satisfied).

Replace Heavier Fare with Vegetables

Portobello mushrooms make great "burgers," or how about a cauliflower-rice mushroom vegetable burger? Swapping veggies for heavier fare can help keep recipes lighter (and *simple!*), especially during the summer heat, and amp up the satiety and nutrition factors of traditionally fiberless recipes.

Celebrate Good Times, Come On!

Celebrating someone else's joy or your own is great, but the food and drink components of celebrating can be tough to navigate in terms of preserving your healthy habits. Looking forward to weekend celebrations—the multiple-day scenarios of having a grand old time—whether you're whooping it up in Nashville at a bachelorette party, raging at your cousin's bar mitzvah, nervously prepping for your own wedding (mazel!), or just going out (hey, you're single and ready to mingle!)?

- **Take time to curate your dream (diet).** Start by thinking about what would help you achieve your end goal of presenting what you feel is the best version of yourself on the big day, whether that's a wedding, reunion, vacation, or much-anticipated date. Is there a sport you love, music that always gets you going, or an activity that brings you peace of mind? Starting a new exercise plan or trying out a new workout class is a great way to feel energized and motivated, but make sure you leave class feeling good and not miserable. When it comes to your diet, it's fine to try to make healthy choices, but don't suffer; downloading a meal-tracking app and cooking some nutritious recipes at home are both reasonable, actionable things you can start right away. These actions will help you work toward your health goals in a safe and effective way—and may even help you stick with your newfound plan once the big day has come and gone.
- **Be realistic about your (weight-loss) vision.** Let's say, for example, you decided your goal was to learn to speak French: You wouldn't start by conjugating verbs in the past tense! In the same way, losing weight at a rapid rate can backfire and lead to rapid weight gain! So how do you avoid this?
  - Think about setting quantifiable weight-loss goals for each week until the big day—ones that you know you can reasonably have a chance of attaining regardless of your insane work schedule, last-minute emergencies, or travel.
  - Start small and keep it simple: Complete meal and snack planning for the week during the weekend before, which will help you factor

in the treats that are a normal part of parties and celebrations that will occur along the way.

- Maintain reasonable boundaries on your to-do list to avoid burn-out (remember: half marathons before full marathons!). In other words, "I'm going to buy ingredients to cook *three* nights [not every night] this week," and "I'm going to make it to *one* kickboxing class [not three kickboxing classes] this week."

■ **Resist the urge to eliminate a food group.** Personal pet peeve about traditional diets (besides everything): There's always a lot of focus on what you *can't* do rather than what you *can* do! (Ah, yes, readers! There's a method to the madness behind the word *more*!) You can help yourself change that thinking by, first, changing your language. Instead of saying things like "cut down on," "eliminate," or "don't eat," switch up the narrative to concentrate on what you *can* do on your new healthy eating plan: "Double up on colorful fruits and veg-gies," "Have [1 ounce of] chocolate for dessert tonight," and "Drink one glass of red with dinner." Using words that remind you of happy, enjoyable foods and activities that will *also* help you on your weight-loss journey will keep you sane (and looking forward to the occasion you're preparing for in the first place!).

■ **Get hard-core about vegging out.** The one thing you *should* get seri-ous about is adding more vegetables (and fruits) to every meal of your day. The more you're able to *add* these foods to everything you eat, the easier it will be to displace the "junk" (e.g., sweetened bever-ages, cookies, cakes, candy, and all the other extra-processed stuff). What this looks like: extra veggies on an omelet at breakfast; snack-ing on precut veggies with hummus, yogurt dressing, or nut butter; stuffing as many veggies as possible into your sandwich at lunch; and trying out one new veggie at dinner this week. One added benefit of veggies and fruit, besides taking the place of less nutritious foods, is that they're filled with bloat-busting minerals that can help you natu-rally shed extra weight you might be holding on to from high-sodium foods or day-to-day water retention.

■ **Amp up the hydration.** By adding vegetables and fruits to your meals and snacks, you'll also help meet your hydration needs. In addition to sipping unsweetened coffee and tea, add fruit (melon, berries, and citrus) to water and seltzer for extra flavor and nutritional benefits. Aim for at least 8–10 cups of fluids per day.

- **Snack (on the right things) with abandon.** The key to weight-loss success is eating frequently—at least every three to four hours. Snacks should be a filling combo of protein and fiber (no less than 3 g of each) and be made from real, whole foods (e.g., fruit and nuts; unsweetened snack mixes; toast with nut butter; bagel thin with cottage cheese and tomatoes).

- **Be the master of multitasking.** Need to go over the agenda for next week's meeting? On a conference call with a caterer? Do it while you're on a walk (or even a run—albeit, a slow run!).

And if you're really adventurous and seriously pressed for time: Walk and talk *on your way to a workout*. Scheduling your daily responsibilities around a workout can help you complete *both*—without feeling the guilt of "I should be doing *more*!" Turning a specific part of your day into a combo of "me" time and checking a few items off your to-do list can help relieve stress across the board.

Staying Accountable Is Positive; Getting Competitive Is Not

It might be irritating to be at dinner with a friend who waves away the bread basket and says, "No thanks, I'm losing weight for *my wedding*." But on the flip side, and to your friend's credit, if *no one* knows you're trying to make healthier choices, it's harder to stick with them! People who are accountable to some*thing* or some*one* (e.g., a training schedule, a friend, or a registered dietitian) tend to stay on track and make long-term changes that *stick*. Your accountability partner could even be your personal journal (that no one ever reads!) or a friend who lives overseas that you see only twice a year. Research has shown that just the act of writing down what you're eating *while* you're eating it (aka a food journal) can help you lose weight because of the accountability aspect. Accountability *works* as a weight-loss motivator.

One note of caution, however: Emotions run high in preparing for weddings as it is, so be wary of toxic frenemies who try to lure you into a pre-wedding weight-loss competition instead of supporting you and cheering you on.

Reminder: It's a Marathon, Not a Sprint

If you ignore all else, keep this one nugget of information in mind: The most important thing you can do when you're starting a new eating plan of any kind is to give yourself permission to mess up once in a while. It happens. Life is too short to *constantly* count calories, *always* choose the "healthiest" thing on the menu, or worry yourself into a guilt frenzy about that burger (and fries) you ate during the bachelorette weekend. If you overindulge, or lose track for a day, a week, or even a month, you can start over. Keep in mind that these events—be it your wedding, a birthday party, a reunion, or your kid's bar mitzvah—are joyous, beautiful, momentous occasions that you deserve to celebrate fully—without any regrets. Don't let a slice of cake stop you from loving every moment of it!

Season's ~~Greetings~~ Eatings!

The main question I'm asked around the holidays is some version of "How can I avoid overeating?" Thanksgiving, Hanukkah, Christmas, Kwanzaa… Celebrating any of these holidays includes food and treats that traditionally don't enter your rotation too often. But there are ways in which you can be proactive to guard against a complete takedown via peppermint bark. Add a little more reason to the season with some of these ideas:

PUMPKIN SPICE SEASON

There's a strange phenomenon between Labor Day and Black Friday, in which everyone, everywhere seems to just somehow "forget" that pumpkins are a vegetable, and supermarkets, menus, and even drugstores are suddenly riddled with an influx of pumpkin spice–flavored products: everything from coffee to muffins to ice cream to cereal to even dog treats. The good news about this is that the pumpkin itself is a *vegetable* (and a super nutritious one, too!). One cup of pumpkin contains more vitamin A than a cup of kale, more potassium than a banana, and more fiber than ½ cup of quinoa. But since the pumpkin *spice*–flavored products also contain a significantly less nutritious blend of nutmeg, cinnamon, sugar, and orange food coloring, they deserve a second review of the ingredients list before you throw them into your shopping cart or place an order:

- Look for pumpkin spice products that list actual pumpkin as the first or second ingredient (for yogurts, ice cream, baked goods, and snack bars that's a must; for cereals and spreads, a few ingredients down is okay on occasion). As long as the first ingredient is a *real food* and not a sneaky name for sugar or some synthetic form of "protein blend," you're good to go.
- Check that your pick has as few ingredients and grams of sugar as possible (single-digit grams of sugar per serving is always a good gauge). Dairy and fruit-containing products may be a little higher (aim to cap yogurt at 12 g of sugar per serving) since these contain naturally occurring sugar.
- Seriously, skip the sugary beverages whenever possible. Yes, that *does include* the pumpkin spice latte. Instead, add 2 tablespoons of half-and-half to your regular cup of joe; sprinkle in pumpkin pie spice to your heart's content; sweeten as you normally would; and serve with a cinnamon stick for an easy festive treat (but with lower sugar and lower calories).

Here's a thought: You can enjoy pumpkin year-round (with or without the "spice")! This powerhouse vegetable can easily be added to:

- Sauces: Substitute pumpkin for half the cheese in sauce. This is the best trick of all time because if you're seasoning the sauce with a little extra flavor (garlic, onion, and even a tablespoon or two of Parmesan—an extra flavorful hard cheese) the pumpkin will add a more creamy quality without sacrificing flavor.
- Greek yogurt or cottage cheese with cinnamon, pumpkin pie spice, and a sprinkle of graham cracker (look, everyone! It's pie!).

- Greek yogurt with cinnamon, honey, pumpkin pie spice, and a cinnamon stick (you're fancy! And it's a sweet dip that you can serve with apple or pear slices!).
- Breakfast of any kind: Making waffles? Add pumpkin puree. Making any type of bready baked good? Add pumpkin. Working on your kid's math homework? X + Y + pumpkin puree = problems, solved.

Holiday Eating Survival Plan

Here's the thing about the holidays: The actual *meal* (e.g., Thanksgiving, Christmas, your birthday, your kid's birthday, your parent's birthday...you get the idea) *cannot* cause real, substantial weight gain (yep—even if you eat your weight in pie!). In fact, it's actually all of the things we eat in the days and weeks *before* and *after* the main treat-yourself-palooza that keep us in a steady weight-gaining zone, most commonly seen nationwide from pre-Thanksgiving straight through spring break. (Yes, RDs like me do this, too!) But what takes us from the traditional holiday indulgence to the season-long all-you-can-eat buffet is lack of preparation. Where to start? With this super simple, streamlined to-do list that'll help you spring back from any or many indulgent days of eating and drinking.

1. Have a post-holiday game plan.

Start by making a game plan. When you're shopping for the feast, grab a few extra essentials that will *really* matter when you're fresh out of leftovers: Eggs; fresh or frozen veggies (for omelets); Greek yogurt; fruit, hummus, nut butter; and canned salmon or tuna (for adding protein to salads) can help you automate the "get-back-to-business" eating habits.

2. Eat more, not less.

It may sound counterintuitive, but the first step to getting back on track after a days' long food coma is actually to *eat*! (You know this one already!) You've skipped breakfast and lunch, so you're ready to take down a whole ham by dinner; you ignored all of my (very sound!) advice and survived on naked salad leaves…until you got to the office bake sale and took down a whole brownie tin, etc. A foolproof trick to try: Make it your mission to go back to the basics: eat breakfast, eat regularly (no skipping), stay satisfied (not just full), and be mindful of your willpower sh*t starters. Seriously committed snackers, chew on this: Set a "snack alarm" on your phone to go off every 3.5 hours, and lend Bob from accounting your noise-canceling headphones if he has a problem with it. (*No need to be a Grinch, Bob!*)

3. Snack for satiety.

Snack recap: Aim to make all of your snacks between 150 and 250 calories and a combo of a fiber-packed carb (e.g., whole grains, fruit, veggies) and lean protein (e.g., eggs, legumes, nuts, part-skim dairy). Some good snack combos would include an apple and a tablespoon of peanut butter; a slice of cheese and a pear; 2–3 tablespoons of hummus with chopped veggies and about 15 whole-grain crackers…you get the point. We often need a little extra produce (shocking!) to help us just feel like we're doing something extra beneficial for ourselves, especially if we feel like we've gone "off-track." And of course, it's the combo of these nutrients that helps to keep you satisfied—not just *full*.

4. Skip the beverages.

Ease up on mocha lattes there, Scotty! We'll talk more about sugary bevs in the next few chapters, but whenever you feel like you need a reset, this is arguably the easiest place to start for many of us: Make all of your beverages non-nutritive, meaning that you're switching from vanilla latte to black coffee and from regular soda to flavored sparkling water, and keeping alcohol to a minimum (max out at a drink per day of clears only: vodka/tequila/gin with soda or water).

Key sneaky calorie culprits: Sugar-sweetened beverages (like juice, or sweetened coffee and tea), dressings, gravies and sauces, sweetened dried fruit, and condiments (like mayo on sandwiches and cooking oil in stir-fries) can rack up calories—quickly. Your best bet for expediting weight loss: Stick with unsweetened beverages only (many of us are still consuming *way* more than we think from cocktail mixes and sweetened coffee beverages). Making some calculated, empowered choices when it comes to what you eat can help you figure out the things you know you can do without while avoiding that "deprived" feeling that occurs when you've eliminated something, restricted a nutrient or a food group, and ultimately paved the path for an unintentional "screw it!" situation.

The number one way to nip any potential diet-derailing damage in the bud: Don't kick yourself for indulging. Yes, we are all humans who sometimes celebrate a little too hard, eat pie for a few meals in a row, and bathe in mashed potatoes for a little longer than we "should." And yes, we *all* (especially *us*, ladies!) have a knack for beating ourselves up when we're imperfect or things don't go exactly as planned. Resist the urge to throw yourself a pity party, because *that's* the key to improving your health and staying on track for the long-term.

YOUR COMPLETE GUIDE TO PARTY EATING

Before

- Eat breakfast: eggs/egg sandwich, peanut butter, piece of fruit, whole-grain toast, and unsweetened Greek yogurt with fruit are high in protein but also fiber-filled. Your biggest mistake would be attempting to "save calories" for later, because that can backfire twofold: (1) You'll feel the effects of any alcohol you drink faster, and (2) you'll be even hungrier later.
- Hydrate early; hydrate *often*! All throughout the day leading up to the party, and especially a 16-ounce glass one hour to thirty minutes before you head out.
- Also in that time window: Your pregame snack. Pack it with protein and fiber (like nuts and seeds, unsweetened yogurt, or whole-grain toast with peanut butter)—150 to 250 calories, one hour before the event.

During

- Build a better plate: veggies, veggies, and more veggies. Wherever you are—fresh, grilled, skewered—even with dip (which often gets a bad rap). Veggies will help you fill up on fiber and are high in water content, so you'll also help stave off a hangover later on. Once you've substantially filled up on the good stuff, you can go in for a serving of something more decadent (savory or sweet!). Check out the chicken, beef, or salmon appetizers. Another great choice: the raw bar (when available).

- #protip: Why dive into a plate of stale saltine crackers and cheese that you could have anytime at home?! Choose two of the foods you love the *most* at any event, or ones that you wouldn't normally buy for yourself. You're better off indulging in a couple of things you don't get to enjoy as often, such as charcuterie and cheese with fruit, rather than filling up on standard fare.

After

- Chug (water). At least 16 ounces right away when you get home. You can prep ahead before the party with a bike bottle (about 24 ounces—even better!) of water, club soda, or a diet ginger ale/unsweetened ginger tea.
- If you're still hungry: Choose foods that are available in a single serving—individually wrapped cheese, bag of nuts or seeds, roasted chickpeas or bean-based snacks, or the ½ sandwich (like turkey on whole-grain bread) left over from lunch. All of these foods are high in potassium, magnesium, and calcium, which can help balance electrolytes lost while partying. Most important: Skip high-fat foods (ahem, the fried stuff) and things like tomatoes, chocolate, and peppermint (no candy canes post-midnight!); all of these are reflux-inducing foods, so if you're susceptible to GERD, avoid these within ninety minutes of bedtime.
- The next day: Drink coffee! Tons of research supports the mental alertness benefits of drinking coffee first thing in the morning, so anywhere from 300 to 400 milligrams of caffeine per day (400 mg = about 1 venti [20 ounces] Starbucks coffee) is A-OK (based on personal tolerance, though, so go with whatever works for you). Raise your blood sugar levels with real fruit, not juice or a little "hair of the dog." Juice spikes blood sugar, which can lead you right into the arms of a major crash; more alcohol just delays the effects of an already-horrific hangover.

#protip

Holiday Swaps (That You Can Use All Year)

Mashed potatoes: Use mashed high-fiber, super-low-cal cauliflower for half of your mashed potato dish. At 150 calories per head, you can eat this weight-loss flower in heaping portions, and when it's substituted for heavier fare, you'll easily cut your calorie intake by *half*. If you're doing this with sweet potatoes, don't forget to add a little pumpkin puree for flavor—more fiber for fewer calories is a good swap!

Sour cream, dips, and dressings: Try 2% or nonfat Greek yogurt instead of sour cream. It's lower in saturated fat and higher in protein and will cut calories without skimping on that creamy deliciousness you crave this time of year. Mix the yogurt with spices like onion and garlic powders, chili flakes, and chives for a healthier take on dips and dressings.

Apple pie: Try a baked apple with cinnamon, nutmeg, and a drizzle of almond butter, topped with cinnamon graham cracker crumbs (from half of a graham cracker sheet). This dessert feels decadent since you'll get the creaminess of the nut butter (add some cacao nibs or top with dark chocolate chips for an extra hit of indulgence). Because baked apples are made in single servings (one apple per person), they're a smart swap for pie since you're not reaching back in for another sliver of pie. Plus, crumbled graham cracker instead of pie crust? Genius!

Potato latkes: Substitute butternut squash, parsnips, or carrots for half the potatoes. You'll add antioxidants and fiber, and the updated take on a traditional Hanukkah favorite will keep guests guessing!

Stuffing: Try a whole grain instead of bread in your usual stuffing recipe this year. Quinoa, buckwheat, teff, millet, or amaranth will add a nuttier flavor and filling fiber to cut cravings and fill you up faster.

6

Grocery Shopping Gives Me Anxiety!

After this chapter, you will...

- understand marketing claims and third-party verifications on packaged foods;
- read a Nutrition Facts label like a boss;
- shop the supermarket with nutrition know-how; and
- know how to write a shopping list that will save you money, time, and headaches.

Confession: I *live* for the supermarket. I like being there so much that I'll often seek out random, unknown megastores, farmer's markets, national food chains, roadside markets, and completely unassuming gas station mini-marts just about *everywhere* I go. (It's *fieldwork*, you know?!) I get a little *frisson* of excitement just from walking up and down each aisle, seeing which products are new versus what has stood the test of time, and randomly exclaiming, "What a load of bs!" when I see overpriced, overpromising items masquerading as health foods.

For many of my clients, however, grocery shopping is a huge source of stress in their regular lives. When it comes to navigating the supermarket, there are so many options, which generate so many questions and so much confusion, that food shopping can incite a sense of dread comparable to what you might feel about going to the dentist (for a root canal).

The good news? It doesn't *have* to be that way! Stick with me, and you'll never wonder *What do I do with all of this food?!* or *How can it be that I went to the grocery store and I still have nothing I want for dinner?!* again. I'll also arm you with all of the tools you need to cut through the fog of misleading labels, confusing portion sizes, impulse shopping, and the other anxiety-producing factors that can make food shopping a drag.

Option Overload: The Beauty (and the Beast) of a Free-Market Society

Imagine this: You walk into the supermarket, innocently looking to pick up a few items, including some hot cereal, which you've been meaning to add to your pantry. You reach the cereal aisle after adding Windex and brownie tins to your cart, only to find that there are approximately 1.2 *gazillion* cereals (give or take…). A large portion of those seem to be different types of oatmeal, and they range from "plain" to "blueberry" to "steel-cut" to "quick" to "gluten-free" and on and on. Some are available in a multipack while others are in a clear pack and others in a canister. There's muesli, overnight muesli, and overnight oats, and you can buy those overnight versions in plain or apple or peaches and cream. Plus, there are the claims of "more protein," "more fiber," and "50% less sugar"; there's also "no sugar added" and "sugar-free" (and those two appear to be different, for reasons [still] elusive to you). And you can *forget it* if you even thought you might find a time-honored classic, like *farina*.

(Anyone still eating farina…? Cool.)

There are so many *choices* to make that you basically develop decision fatigue and wind up just getting a box of regular, *cold* cereal you know you like with a cartoon animal on it.

Your inner monologue in the dairy aisle *alone* can be enough to make you throw in the towel and drive to Carvel. I know it can feel (and sound) something like this:

Hmm…okay, milk is first on my list. Let me start here. Wait, what kind of milk, though? Skim and nonfat milk are the same thing, right? Right. Wait, I should get cream for coffee, though. Fat-free cream? Definitely getting this. Isn't cream made from fat, though? How do you even make fat-free cream?! Whatever, it's fat-free, it's cream, it's organic, and I'm not asking questions. Wait, it's $6.99?! Maybe I'll pass. Okay—some yogurt would be good. Wow—there are so many Greek yogurts over here! And what is "Skyr" yogurt? I probably should *try it. But I've also read that you shouldn't buy stuff you can't pronounce, and I have no idea how to actually say that word aloud. Why do these yogurts say "organic," but these say "milk from grass-fed cows"? And this one is "natural strawberry." I just don't know. Wait, but what about these—they're naturally flavored and Moana is on the front and my nieces love Moana. I'm totally buying this yogurt (best aunt ever). Okay, but what about the milk…*

(Food shopping is so hard, right?! But it's about to get much easier—I promise!)

Toss, Keep, Buy: Your Kitchen Redesign

Let's bring in some advice from the queen of all organizing gurus, Marie Kondo. (We've never met, but in case this book is ever translated into Japanese, well, *Arigatō gozaimashita*, Marie!)

Kondo-ing your kitchen is pretty simple from a nutritional standpoint—but it takes a little self-evaluation first. When I do this one-on-one with clients, I typically start with getting rid of what I like to call "assorted hoardeds" (basically, stuff you've accumulated from random holidays and family events, like Easter eggs even though it's July, matzoh in the back of a cabinet, expiration dated "January 2003," etc.) and college cuisine (like that ramen you've been stocking up on since your dorm-room days). Then we tackle your personal trigger foods (I'll explain further below); uncover sneaky sources of added sugar that are "hiding" in your cupboard or refrigerator (spooky!); and expose the items masquerading as health food—which you bought because they seemed or claimed to be "healthy" but are actually either total garbage or something you're never going to eat (so, as Marie would say, time to let it go). Since I won't be joining you in your kitchen, I recommend putting on a playlist you love, grabbing some garbage bags, and rolling up your sleeves—this part will be positively freeing!

What to Toss:

- Thanksgiving leftovers/Halloween candy.
- White-flour pastries, biscuits, buns, bagels, crackers.
- Tempting condiments that can double as finger food when you want it badly enough (whipped topping, cheese dip, icing, frosting, sour cream…you get the point).

- College cuisine (ramen, frozen or pantry mac 'n cheese, chips, soda, sweet/sad cereal, sweet/sad pretzels, fake cheese crackers).
- Deli meat (packaged, processed, and/or plastic-wrapped meat).
- Protein that you refer to as "protein": powders, bars, shakes, supplements (I know they were expensive! But now you've read chapter 3 and they've got to go . . . new year, new you and all!).
- "Veggie" chips, sweetened dried fruit, and anything else you bought under the influence of a "health halo."

Use these terms to determine what to buy, *when*, and what to toss *right now*. This chart will give you a rundown on expiration dates: What you might *think* they mean isn't what they actually mean:

Sell by: This is a guideline for your retailer to use in restocking shelves.

Use by: Consumer guideline, but doesn't necessarily mean much if the product is not perishable.

Best by: Indicator of freshness, not safety or spoilage.

What to Keep:

We'll cover more on what to keep and why below, but here are some items you may have stored at home that can be put to good use—don't toss 'em just yet!

- Butter/cooking oil
- Spices
- Canned, frozen, or pouched: beans, lentils, chickpeas, peas, pumpkin, artichokes/artichoke hearts, tomatoes
- Frozen fruits and vegetables
- Nuts, seeds, blends, and butters
- Unsweetened fruit: canned or dried
- 100 percent whole grains

What to Know Before You Go Shopping: The Silent Influencers of Your Grocery Cart

The myriad of claims related to health and agricultural practices make it almost impossible to navigate the food store shelves with confidence minus some higher level of knowledge in both nutrition and advertising. What you "know" about nutrition-related information may feel inadequate but at the same time contradictory to some of the theories that are pervasive in the current nutrition landscape.

The trouble is that there are many different organizations in both the public and the private sectors with a financial stake in defining what is considered healthy for the general public. Before we get into how you can start gaining more confidence in shopping for food, I think it would help to take a closer look at some of the primary ways that the health value of our food is determined. In my experience, it's these variables that play a significant role in determining what winds up in your grocery cart (and ultimately, your mouth):

- Varying interpretations of scientific research
- Federal guidelines and policy as a result of these interpretations
- Communication (and miscommunication) of that research
- The resulting development, marketing, and distribution of food

Let's talk about how to put these variables into the appropriate context *before* you start food shopping.

The United States Department of Agriculture (USDA) and the Department of Health and Human Services (HHS) join forces every five years to publish the *Dietary Guidelines for Americans* (*DGA*), a reference guide for the food industry, public health recommendations, and government programs (like SNAP, WIC, and school food). You may have seen or heard of portions of these guidelines in their consumer-friendly formats: the Food Guide Pyramid (introduced in 1992); MyPyramid (as of 2005); and the current tool, MyPlate (introduced in 2010). Historically, these guidelines have been intended to help the American public meet nutrient requirements to promote better health, but the most recent guidelines emphasize the idea of "healthier eating patterns," with the goal of helping us all create a better eating plan overall without fixating on specific nutrient requirements.

The *DGA* is powerful for one highly important reason: Food and agriculture industries account for 21.4 *million jobs* in the U.S. and contribute $992 *billion* to the U.S. GDP. This includes food companies, agricultural workers, and anyone else who makes a living off any aspect of food production— from farming and growing to research and development of food products, to packaging and distribution, to the marketing and advertising of it all. Since these stakeholders care deeply about how the *DGA* are communicated to consumers *and* how that impacts their product development, it is, to put it bluntly, kind of a *big deal*.

As noted above, the USDA and HHS release the *DGA* in a collaborative effort. These two major government bodies vet for the safety of pretty much everything (well, *mostly* everything) we could possibly ingest. The USDA is primarily focused on agriculture, of course, while the HHS is primarily focused on human, animal, and pet health. There is also a government-appointed advisory committee made up of experts in different areas of nutrition research, though with nongovernmental backgrounds, who review the dietary guidelines of years past and make suggested updates based on new literature that's been published in the five years since the release of the most recent edition of the *DGA*. Each term, the administrative lead is charged with appointing the committee, and that responsibility alternates every five years between the HHS and the USDA.

Why should you care about any of this? Well, because (a) statistically speaking, you may very well *work in some aspect of the food industry*, and (b) the politics behind the scenes of the DGA provides a fascinating framework that's crucial to understanding *why* news and media coverage on the food industry is so conflicting and disjointed, creating the optimal environment in which diet fads and elimination diets rise and *thrive*.

The Dietary Guidelines Advisory Committee is *discretionary*, meaning that it's established by either the U.S. Secretary of Health or the U.S. Secretary of Agriculture, depending on the year. In other words, regardless of how many changes or how few changes are *actually made to the guidelines* each term, they will always be viewed as *offensive* to *someone* because of the rotating administrative lead.

When it's the USDA's turn, critics raise concerns that the guidelines are too favorable toward agricultural interests and don't adequately address industry concerns. When the HHS leads, critics raise concerns that the guidelines are too favorable toward public health needs and don't adequately satisfy the needs of farming and food production. It's these opposing views that contribute to an overall disillusionment with what we commonly know to be true about sound nutrition advice, and, rather, pave a comfortable, welcoming path for "diet culture" to make its way into our multimedia newsfeeds.

Let me tell you a little story about tree nuts.

Every five years when the *Dietary Guidelines for Americans* is published, the massive, research-heavy, info-dense document is accompanied by a statement that summarizes the key takeaways from each of the recommendations. The Dietary Guidelines Executive Summary in 2010 made a clear statement that still stands true today: The American diet is high in sodium, and we should cut back to 2,300 mg/day (1,500 mg for those at risk for heart disease). Interestingly, the guidelines went on to make recommendations about which foods Americans should eat more of. One recommendation states very clearly, "Eat unsalted nuts and seeds."

Sounds reasonable, right? Reasonable, sure. Logical? Not quite.

Most salted nut products have 140 mg or less of sodium per a standard 1-ounce serving size. Go to any deli, grocery store, even Amazon, and you'll notice this right off the bat. In fact, many salted nut products have earned the American Heart Association "seal" for heart-healthy benefits.

That's because the Food and Drug Administration and the American Heart Association consider 140 mg and under to be the standard guideline for products stating "low sodium" on their labeling. The difference, then, between 0 mg and 140 mg in a serving of nuts is pretty negligible for most healthy adults. By contrast, 1 cup of the magical cure-all elixir otherwise known as ~~SOUP~~ bone broth contains about 300 mg in the *reduced-sodium version*! (The regular version contains about 480 mg/cup.)

See what happened? The USDA/HHS wanted to say, "Cut back on sodium," but when the guidelines were written, they made an enormous boo-boo by writing "Eat *unsalted* nuts." Bottom line: Of all the things in the world that are loaded with sodium, salted nuts are the least of our worries! To this day, I hear of friends, colleagues, family members, clients, and coworkers alike buying nuts labeled "unsalted" and then not eating them because, in case you haven't indulged: They taste more like woodchips than snacks.

Anyone whose livelihood depends in any way on the production, distribution, and sale of food (or a product, technology, or material that is involved in food production) feels that they have a stake in the language used in the *DGA*. This is the major reason why many feel that it requires federal regulation and many others feel that the federal government should stay out of it.

In order to combat the perception of bias, the *DGA* will sometimes put out helpful summary guides such as the one on the next page.

See what they did here? When the *DGA* tells you what *you should eat*, they give specific food names: "fruits," "oils," "vegetables." When the *DGA* tells you what to limit, they name specific *nutrients*: "saturated fat," "sodium," "added sugar."

That's some politically correct language if I've ever seen it. The *DGA* is carefully attempting to play a moderator's role of being both deferential to industry (not calling out specific foods produced by major corporations) *and* doing justice to the scientific evidence, which suggests that Americans *overconsume* these three nutrients.

As we hear more conflicting opinions, we lose an increased amount of faith in nutrition recommendations and consensus-driven nutrition knowledge, something that ultimately allows scientific half-truths to become a large part of our own cultural vernacular. So what do you *do* about it? Now that you know one major reason why it exists, you can *ignore* inflammatory one-offs and inconsistent language! As Queen Marie might add, "Thank you and good-bye!"

(This is so *liberating*, no?!)

Here's what you need to know. Contrary to hyperbolic headlines (*Time* magazine's 2016 cover stating, "Eat Butter," anyone?), the *DGA* has always had a consistent, consensus-driven backbone about macronutrient

Key Recommendations

Consume a healthy eating pattern that accounts for all foods and beverages within an appropriate calorie level.

A healthy eating pattern includes:[2]

- A variety of vegetables from all of the subgroups—dark green, red and orange, legumes (beans and peas), starchy, and other

- Fruits, especially whole fruits

- Grains, at least half of which are whole grains

- Fat-free or low-fat dairy, including milk, yogurt, cheese, and/or fortified soy beverages

- A variety of protein foods, including seafood, lean meats and poultry, eggs, legumes (beans and peas), and nuts, seeds, and soy products

- Oils

A healthy eating pattern limits:

- Saturated fats and *trans* fats, added sugars and sodium

Key Recommendations that are quantitative are provided for several components of the diet that should be limited. These components are of particular public health concern in the United States, and the specified limits can help individuals achieve healthy eating patterns within calorie limits:

- Consume less than 10 percent of calories per day from added sugars[3]
- Consume less than 10 percent of calories per day from saturated fats[4]
- Consume less than 2,300 milligrams (mg) per day of sodium[5]
- If alcohol is consumed, it should be consumed in moderation—up to one drink per day for women and up to two drinks per day for men—and only by adults of legal drinking age.[6]

[2] Definitions for each food group and subgroup are provided throughout the chapter and are compiled in Appendix 3. USDA Food Patterns: Healthy U.S.-Style Eating Pattern.

[3] The recommendation to limit intake of calories from added sugars to less than 10 percent per day is a target based on food pattern modeling and national data on intakes of calories from added sugars that demonstrate the public health need to limit calories from added sugars to meet food group and nutrient needs within calorie limits. The limit on calories from added sugars is not a Tolerable Upper Intake Level (UL) set by the Institute of Medicine (IOM). For most calorie levels, there are not enough calories available after meeting food group needs to consume 10 percent of calories from added sugars and 10 percent of calories from saturated fats and still stay within calorie limits.

[4] The recommendation to limit intake of calories from saturated fats to less than 10 percent per day is a target based on evidence that replacing saturated fats with unsaturated fats is associated with reduced risk of cardiovascular disease. The limit on calories from saturated fats is not a UL set by the IOM. For most calorie levels, there are not enough calories available after meeting food group needs to consume 10 percent of calories from added sugars and 10 percent of calories from saturated fats and still stay within calorie limits.

[5] The recommendation to limit intake of sodium to less than 2,300 mg per day is the UL for individuals ages 14 years and older set by the IOM. The recommendations for children younger than 14 years of age are the IOM age- and sex-appropriate ULs (see Appendix 7. Nutritional Goals for Age-Sex Groups Based on Dietary Reference Intakes and Dietary Guidelines Recommendations).

[6] It is not recommended that individuals begin drinking or drink more for any reason. The amount of alcohol and calories in beverages varies and should be accounted for within the limits of healthy eating patterns. Alcohol should be consumed only by adults of legal drinking age. There are many circumstances in which individuals should not drink, such as during pregnancy. See Appendix 9. Alcohol for additional information.

(Adapted from "Key Recommendations: The U.S. Dietary Guidelines for Americans, 2015–2020." https://health.gov /dietaryguidelines/2015/guidelines/chapter-1/key-recommendations/, accessed September 2018.)

composition (protein, fat, and carbs) and is consistent with all other major nutrition and public health recommendations around the globe. New data support similar consensus, with updates in language based on specific areas of study (though many in the nutrition community could have told you *all about the benefits of eating the whole egg* ten-plus *years ago*. But I digress.)

In fact, a study published in 2018 by the *Journal of the American Medical Association* showed that while both low-carb and low-fat diets can "work" for weight loss, focusing on real, whole foods is the most impactful way to lose weight. On further analysis, what was the calorie breakdown of those 600-plus study participants' diet? The standard 50-20-30. What's more—the American Heart Association has stayed consistent with their recommendation that 30 percent of total calories come from fat in their Therapeutic Lifestyle Changes diet, designed for people with heart disease, and the American Diabetes Association bases their publication *Choose Your Foods: Exchange List for Diabetics* on 50 percent of total calories coming from carbohydrates. Both of these diets have a long-standing reputation of being "low-fat" or "low-carb," despite the fact that upon closer look, they're completely consistent with the *Dietary Guidelines for Americans*, and both have a tremendous amount of supporting evidence to show that they "work" in helping to treat their respective disease focus.

All things considered, though: The USDA and HHS do a pretty good job as far as I'm concerned. They're responsible for reviewing population data, human biological science information, agricultural chemistry developments, and constantly evolving research on environmental concerns, and then coming up with their *own guidelines and recommendations* regarding what's best for the American population.

In the end, one simple fact sums up the entirety of the controversy: The term *healthy* is subjective, and, therefore, there are lots of different opinions on both the definition of "good health" and what it takes to achieve it. The science behind health-promoting nutritional composition hasn't actually changed all that much. But the evolution of the food industry and the ubiquitous forms of media that reign over the communication of health guidelines have unnecessarily complicated the message—and now's the time to take back that message and take real action.

So let's get going, shall we?

Forget Everything You Know

Nutrition Labels

Nutrition Facts labels are solely managed by the FDA (an HHS division), meaning that the labels you see on food products are not related to the USDA's MyPlate or the *Dietary Guidelines for Americans*. The Nutrition Facts label uses serving sizes that we *are likely to be eating*, not serving sizes that we *should be eating* (what the *DGA* recommends). Throughout the history of the *DGA* and consumer graphics, different calorie levels have been set to provide Americans with more specific recommendations based on a variety of background information, but they do all hover around the 2,000-calorie mark.

While 2,000 calories may *sound* like a high number to some people and a low number to others, it's *really* subjective. Estimating your energy requirements can be done by using some super complicated calculations, but the simplest way is to use the scientifically validated kilocalories per kilogram method. Multiplying your weight in kilograms by both 25 and 30 will provide you with a calorie-requirement range:

[weight in kilograms] × 25 = lower end of your calorie range

[weight in kilograms] × 30 = upper end of your calorie range

A generally healthy adult female who weighs 140 pounds requires 1,590 to 1,909 calories per day to maintain weight. Needless to say, calorie requirements are different for your kids (if you have them); different for your partner (if you have one); and different for your dog, Fido, whose dietary needs are actually ignored by the *DGA* (*shame!*).

In light of what we know about calories, what should you know about serving sizes? That the "serving size" information shown on food packaging labels has a relatively estranged relationship with the "serving sizes" recommended by the *Dietary Guidelines for Americans* on particular food items. So where does that leave you? Don't rely exclusively on serving sizes as for what to choose. I know, I know: I'm throwing out all the rules that you've been following. But guess what—those rules weren't helping you! And if you keep reading, I'm going to give you the information you need to really understand once and for all what is best for your body. And I promise it's going to make a lot more sense and be very delicious.

HOW MANY INGREDIENTS ARE TOO MANY INGREDIENTS?

In chapter 5, I advised you to choose products with as few ingredients as possible. This is a good rule of thumb, but there is a little nuance involved. Let's take something like often-glorified almond milk. Many of us assume that the ingredients in almond milk are just almonds and water. But in fact, it typically has many more than that. Here's a sample label:

ALMOND MILK (FILTERED WATER, ALMONDS), CANE SUGAR, CAL-CIUM CARBONATE, NATURAL FLAVORS, POTASSIUM CITRATE, SEA SALT, SUNFLOWER LECITHIN, GELLAN GUM, VITAMIN A PALMITATE, VITAMIN D2, D-ALPHA-TOCOPHEROL (NATURAL VITAMIN E)

On the other hand, 100 percent whole-grain bread is a nutrient-dense food that can be made with *tons of different types* of whole grains, including amaranth, quinoa, sorghum, whole wheat, oats, buckwheat, and bulgur. So when you read the ingredients list, you might be surprised at how many ingredients are actually in that sandwich vehicle:

ORGANIC WHOLE WHEAT (ORGANIC WHOLE WHEAT FLOUR, ORGANIC CRACKED WHOLE WHEAT), WATER, POWERSEED MIX (ORGANIC WHOLE FLAXSEEDS, ORGANIC GROUND WHOLE FLAXSEEDS, ORGANIC ROLLED OATS, ORGANIC SUNFLOWER SEEDS, ORGANIC PUMPKIN SEEDS, ORGANIC UN-HULLED BROWN SESAME SEEDS, ORGANIC UN-HULLED BLACK SESAME SEEDS), ORGANIC WHEAT GLUTEN, ORGANIC FRUIT JUICES (ORGANIC APPLE, ORGANIC PEAR, ORGANIC PEACH), ORGANIC OAT FIBER, SEA SALT, ORGANIC CULTURED WHOLE WHEAT, YEAST, ORGANIC VINEGAR

The major difference between the almond milk label and the whole-grain bread label? The types of ingredients—not the *number*. The bread has lots more ingredients, but they're all things that *should be* in a wholesome bread (grains, yeast, seeds). But the milk? It contains added sugar and added sodium—ingredients you might not have expected to find in a milk beverage.

Bottom line: We can't always judge a product by the number of ingredients it has. Rather, we have to pay attention to the types of ingredients in order to make a choice that's right for us.

Old Label Versus New Label (2020): Key Differences

Serving Size

The new food label required by the Food and Drug Administration will employ more recently updated RACCs (reference amounts customarily consumed). But if you think that means digging into a whole pint of ice cream is now A-OK with the FDA, think again. (RACC is what you customarily consume, not what you're supposed to consume!) When the updating of the label was first championed by Michelle Obama in 2013, one of the proposed changes was intended to draw the consumer's attention to the number of calories per serving by showing the number in a larger and bolder type. Serving sizes were also updated to reflect changes in how people eat and drink. For instance, a 20-ounce soda is required to be labeled as 1 serving, rather than the old 2.5 servings (figuring 8 ounces per serving). The First Lady's optimistic hope was that the new labels would promote healthier eating through providing better information.

Personally, I'm skeptical of this theory because of current data demonstrating that calorie labeling in general doesn't necessarily translate into behavioral change. The change in serving size information has definite possibilities for doing some good but needs a bit more consumer education behind it in order to really translate into informing our purchases. This is yet another contentious issue among those in the food industry, however (e.g., a sugary 20-ounce soda label now has to show "130%" of the daily value for added sugar).

Ultimately the label update is more of a Band-Aid attempting to cover up a cut that needs stitches—our overall lack of education in nutrition—but luckily we're *here*, getting educated!! (So we don't have to worry about *that* too much!)

Sugar Breakdown

Added sugars differ from naturally occurring sugars you'll find in foods like dairy products (lactose) and fruit (fructose). Since chronic diseases such as heart disease, diabetes, and some cancers have been linked to an excess of added sugars in our food supply, the FDA differentiates these from their more wholesome counterparts (think plain yogurt versus sweetened yogurt) to help consumers avoid consuming more than 10 percent of their total calories in added sugars. (That translates into 150 to 200 calories per day, as part of a 1,500- to 2,000-calorie diet, from 38 to 50 g of added sugars.) We'll explore added sugar more in the pages ahead, but for now, we'll note that the biggest benefit of this delineation is that it can help many of us ID the top sources of added sugar in our diets (sugary beverages and breakfast pastries) so that we can make better informed choices.

Nutrient Content Claims (NCCs)

Something else you'll find on food labels? Nutrient content claims, otherwise known as NCCs. These are claims that brands are legally permitted to make on their labels to highlight a particular nutrient found in a food product.

Nutrient content claims attribute value to the level of a nutrient in the product based on the daily value of a product, using terms such as *free*, *high*, and *low*. The claims can also be used to compare the level of a nutrient in a particular food to the level in another food, using terms such as *more*, *reduced*, and *lite*. Nutrient content claims are usually permitted by the FDA only if they have an associated daily value. For example, frozen potatoes. A product like this would likely be permitted to use the NCC "good source of potassium," because a normal serving provides at least 10 percent of the recommended daily value for the mineral.

The list of nutrients that have been defined by the FDA as eligible for specific content claims is exhaustive, includes a variety of vitamins and minerals, and is frequently updated. For example, the National Academy of Sciences approved the use of a content claim for the nutrient choline in 2015, due to population data suggesting that Americans eat only 10 percent of what we actually need, and biochemical data suggesting this undervalued compound is fairly crucial for better health. Research suggests that consuming more choline (found in foods such as eggs, shrimp, spinach, peanut butter, and lentils) may help to reduce the risk of heart disease; improve cognition (especially in those at risk for Alzheimer's disease); and decrease the risk of nonalcoholic fatty liver disease; and may be essential for proper fetal brain development.

What makes things complicated with NCCs is the fact that each nutrient is unique to food chemistry and also unique to biochemistry. For example, if a product claim says "30% less fat," that *might* be beneficial to you, but it could also mean that the product is *less filling*, *less satisfying*, and, ultimately, a hunger-promoting product (if you're not full, you're bound to keep snacking, right?!). In certain products, the "reduced fat" alternative probably contains something else to boost flavor, and more often than not, that something is *sugar*. Low-fat Oreos, anyone?

FOOD LABELS 101

- "Low" is defined as 5 percent or less of the daily value (DV); "high" is defined as 20 percent or less of the DV. For example: "Low sodium" is defined as 140 mg or less per serving, or 5 percent of the DV per serving.
- The term "good source of..." indicates that a food provides 10 percent or more of the daily value for a certain nutrient. For example: A "good source of fiber" is defined as having at least 3 grams of fiber, or 10 percent of the DV.
- "Excellent source of..." is defined as containing 20 percent or more of the nutrient's DV.

- "Free" means the product must have less than 5 calories per recommended serving; to be labeled "low-calorie," the food must have 40 calories or less per serving.
- A "low-fat" product should be a food that the consumer would generally recognize as a food that is lower in calories and fat than *other average products of its type.* By contrast, when a company uses the terms *light, fewer, less,* or *reduced,* the FDA requires supporting nutritional information from these companies.

Label Reading: The Bottom Line

To make a very long story short: Nutrient content claims *have* a place at the supermarket. But they don't get you all that far in terms of deciding what's right for *you.* When looking at nutrient content claims, it is important to be a smart shopper and look at the back of the package for the Nutrition Facts label and the listed ingredients. Ultimately, a food product can be complete and utter garbage, and have a claim on the packaging that is *super* misleading—especially when it's something you know you've *heard* about, but aren't necessarily sure of the details.

Another lesser-known fact: The FDA allows a 20 percent "range" of error on those labels. *Twenty percent!* If you ate a snack that someone told you contained 600 calories but you later found out the actual calorie count was as low as 500 and as high as 700, wouldn't you feel ever so slightly duped? Now, this information is no cause for alarm (*120 calories is the difference of mostly air, anyway!*).

Marketing Mayhem: The Health Halo Effect

Here's the long and the short of it: *Healthy* is a word we use a *ton,* but there is not a true consensus on its meaning anymore, a fact made obvious by the many different *opinions* about what "healthy" means in the federal government alone.

According to the FDA:

Healthy is an implied nutrient content claim that characterizes a food as having "healthy" levels of total fat, saturated fat, cholesterol and sodium, as defined in the regulation authorizing use of the claim.

Historically, to bear the term *healthy*, the food must contain less than 3 g of total fat, less than 1 g of saturated fat, no more than 480 mg of sodium, and no more than 60 mg of cholesterol per serving. To date, it's been updated to designate foods with a mix of mono- and polyunsaturated fats; and 10 percent or more of the daily value for potassium and/or vitamin D.

In 2015, the FDA was forced to redefine *healthy* on nutrition labels when KIND, a snack bar company, was told their product no longer qualified for the use of this term because of the fat content. KIND fought back, claiming that nuts are a source of nutritious polyunsaturated and monounsaturated fats, and they called out the FDA for using outdated information to support their "healthy" definition.

Much of the buzz on "healthy" food has gotten louder lately. Calling a single food or product "healthy" has become a marketing ploy more than an accurate description. And come to think of it, shouldn't "healthy" describe people, while "nutritious" describes the foods we eat that help to make us healthy?

Trying to make sense of all the nutrition information and claims on food labels and packages these days can be overwhelming. So here's a cheat sheet of some of the most common health-claim terms that you'll see on packaging—consider this your information jungle machete to hack your way to a clearer path of deciding what to actually buy!

Natural: (Definitely) Not a Thing

This sexy-sounding word is thrown around *everywhere*—from food labels to names of markets, retailers, and even cooking schools! But what does *natural* actually mean? Nada. Zip. Zero. Well, actually, the FDA has a shell of a definition for it by proxy of its definition of what is "artificial." Why? Rather than gather twenty-five federal agencies to form one hundred committees on the topic, the FDA realized pretty quickly that the term *natural* is a loaded one, and it's *highly* subjective. When the public comments period opened on the topic (and closed in April 2017), it was clear that some people believe *natural* means "organic"; others believe the term *natural* is synonymous with "vegetables," and overall, people were vitriolic over whether or not genetically modified foods of any kind in any food product should be allowed to use the term. Of course, every industry felt compelled to submit a comment or change the name of their product. Items like soy sauce and potato chips that used soybean oil or stone-ground corn preemptively changed their names, thinking the legislation would err on the side of *natural* meaning "non-GMO" (e.g., Frito-Lay's non-GMO snack line went from being labeled "Natural" to "Simply," preempting a change in legislation).

Non-GMO or Non-GMO Project Verified

Since GMOs (genetically modified organisms) were introduced into the food supply, they have been the subject of a major and heated debate over their health and environmental implications—and the labeling issue is a whole other beast (GMO labeling has been mandated by certain states and became federal law in 2016). In the United States, genetically modified crops are those that have been altered to be resistant to herbicides and pesticides or to produce pesticides themselves, chemicals that protect crops by decreasing the risk of crop-killing viruses and bugs. The two most common *edible* GMO crops worldwide are soybeans and corn—both of which are ubiquitous ingredients of food on supermarket shelves.

The most recent and comprehensive National Academy of Sciences report states that although genetically modified crops may vary in nutritional composition, the variation is no more than what would occur naturally and among non-GMO crops. What's more—since a main concern of genetically modified food is its effects on human health, the report analyzed data from large-scale studies since GMOs entered the food supply (1990s) but did not find any associations with chronic disease incidence and dietary patterns as they relate to genetically engineered crops.

In fact, the use of GMOs has been linked to environmental benefits because less land and less water overall are required to produce GMO crops as compared to those conventionally produced—largely due to the reduced loss of crops to weeds and insects, plus reduced greenhouse gas emissions (since there's a lower frequency of tilling the fields).

But the bottom line is that GMO crops *themselves* do not appear to cause any health harm as they relate to the food we eat. Since there's a tremendous amount of confusion about what GMO crops actually *are* and whether or not they are less nutritious than conventionally grown products of the same type, let's clear this up right now: The biggest issue with GMOs from a nutritional standpoint is the products in which they're a*ctually contained*. Recap: Corn and soybeans are the predominant genetically engineered crops that are *edible, right*? And where are these two items found in surplus in our diets? Highly processed foods loaded with added sugar (corn syrup) and saturated fat (soy-based emulsifiers). Here's where GMO crops are *not* secretly lurking: most *everything else* (and especially not produce, despite inflammatory headlines). There *have* been attempts to create GMO apples and the ilk, but they're not approved for/available on the general consumer market, so the media circus over the whole ordeal is deeply rooted in misinformation and confusion, confounded by marketing and "clickbait" media headlines.

"USDA-Certified Organic" Versus "Made with Organic Ingredients"

Confusing, but true: Organic production is overseen by the USDA because it is an agricultural practice, not a specific nutrition-related practice. It's got its own set of labeling standards, regulations, and third-party verification: 90 percent of the ingredients in a product must be organic in order to be third-party verified and ultimately bear the USDA organic label; 70 percent of the ingredients must be organic in order to use the phrase "made with organic ingredients." Regardless, this agricultural practice wears a diamond-encrusted crown that puts almost all other health halos to shame, doesn't it?! Remember, though: Organic cane sugar is still sugar; organic chocolate is still chocolate; and organic water is still H_2O, but organic products will cost more than their nonorganic forms.

Fair Trade Certified

You'll often find the phrase on coffee and chocolate packaging—two industries in which labor-related concerns have been raised on a global scale. The certification implies that environmental and labor-related standards are met in the production of the product, including just compensation that leads to empowerment of workers involved in the production—but it doesn't signify any nutritional value of a food or food product.

Other Buzzy Product Claims

Locally sourced/carefully sourced: This is undefined, meaning that my candy bar could be locally sourced from the deli across the street (if I want it to be), or your yogurt might be "locally sourced from the dairy farm down the road"! Regardless, it's a discretionary term.

100 percent traceable/single origin: This is undefined by the FDA, but for our purposes the meaning refers to the origin that's original to a specific commodity product, like Parmigiano-Reggiano from Parma, Italy, versus mass-produced powdered Parmesan cheese off the grocery store shelf. Certified high-quality foods from Italy are labeled DOP, while their wines bear such labels as DOC and DOCG. European Union quality agricultural products and foodstuffs are promoted, and their names and production processes protected from imitation by labels designating PDO (protected designation of origin), PGI (protected geographical indication), and TSG (traditional specialties guaranteed). In the United States, the traceability of where the wild fish was caught or what fishery the farmed variety was raised in is important, and we'll discuss that a little more later on.

Health Halos Part Deux: Allergen Flag or Alarmist Marketing?

Gluten-Free

The claims: Gluten-free products are "anti-inflammatory," and they can help you lose weight; the gluten-free diet is a great way to cut carbs, help your arthritis symptoms, and reduce bloating and belly fat. You already know this is *bananas* after reading chapter 1: If you're on a gluten-free diet for anything other than the treatment of celiac disease or a wheat allergy, you might be doing yourself a disservice. Keep in mind that gluten-free food alternatives are not going to help you lose weight—in fact, they can often make you gain weight because the protein (gluten) is removed from nutritious, filling, and high-fiber foods in order to create a more processed, refined-carb, high-sodium, and saturated-fat-filled alternative. One good example is gluten-free pretzels—the gluten-free versions will contain a minimum of 2 grams of saturated fat, while regular pretzels will not contain any saturated fat.

Dairy-Free

Important distinction: Dairy-free doesn't necessarily mean lactose-free, and vice versa. People who eat dairy-free are often allergic to the casein in milk or are vegan or predominantly vegetarian; people who eat lactose-free usually do so because they don't have enough of the enzyme called *lactase*, which is needed to break down lactose, the sugar found in dairy products. The symptoms of both casein allergy and lactose intolerance are sometimes severe gastrointestinal issues, including diarrhea, nausea, cramps, bloating, and gas.

Nut-Free

Products labeled nut-free must be processed in a nut-free facility, say as much on the ingredients list, and use a "contains" statement. According to the FARE (Food Allergy Research and Education) corporation: "All FDA-regulated manufactured food products that contain a 'major food allergen' (milk, wheat, egg, peanuts, tree nuts, fish, crustacean shellfish, and soy) as an ingredient are required by US law to list that allergen on the product label. For tree nuts, fish and crustacean shellfish, the specific type of nut or fish must be listed."

FARE is an amazing resource for anyone with a nut allergy, and their website has some useful food-shopping tips. But since tree-nut allergies are relatively uncommon in their incidence (occurring in less than 1 percent of the U.S. population and between 1 and 6 percent of children) and their symptoms are so severe, I trust this claim is crucial to you if you're already looking for it.

The Claims Decoder

Too many claims are misunderstood. Here is the short list of food examples with sexy claims that aren't all that great for you:

Healthy: Sneaky junk-food examples: breakfast items and pastries like Pop-Tarts, sugary cereals, orange juice, and breakfast breads (all of which might claim, "Healthy choice for the whole family!").

Simple/simply; traditional: These are 2018's new words meaning "natural." You'll see them on the aforementioned potato chips, sauces, dips, and basically any processed food that had used an ingredient in a prior version that might have been subjected to genetic modification (e.g., corn and soybeans).

No sugar added: Sneaky junk-food examples: fruit snacks and smoothies that use "fruit juice concentrate" to get around the FDA labeling law.

All-natural: Sneaky junk-food examples: cookies, candy, chips— your average supermarket snack staples—might be labeled "all natural," as well as veggie chips, granola bars, and cereal. Since the term is left undefined by the FDA, it's still allowed despite the efforts of major food companies to get rid of it.

No artificial sweetener: Lots of yogurt and yogurt drinks make this claim but are loaded up with chicory root fiber, stevia, and inulin—these are not "artificial" by FDA definition, but if you're sensitive to sugar substitutes (and many of us may be unknowingly sensitive), they can upset your GI tract. Plus, if you're cooking with them (e.g., using a plain Greek yogurt made with chicory root), you can expect these to be sweet-tasting rather than savory.

No cholesterol: Sneaky junk-food examples: grains of all kinds— from rice to bagels to whole-grain cereals. This unnecessary claim is still out there...even though the only foods that contain dietary sources of cholesterol are from *animals* (dairy, meat, fish— nothing plant-based should have cholesterol to begin with!). The only ingredients in a potato chip are often potatoes, oil, and salt. So *why oh why* would cholesterol be in there in the first place?! Food companies are still allowed to use "no cholesterol" if the product contains 2 g or more of saturated fat.

Vegan: Sneaky junk-food examples: snack mixes and snack bars. Just because there's a halo around "vegan" diets doesn't mean vegan products are any better for you than options that *aren't* vegan. They're often sugar bombs, also loaded with added saturated fat and sodium. One such culprit is often "coconut oil," which is lauded for its "health benefits," all of which are totally bogus.

Nutrient content claims, while highly regulated by the FDA, tend to highlight one particular positive aspect of a food product and neglect the product's potential downsides. For example, a cookie might be labeled "fat-free" as a marketing strategy, but the packaging won't highlight its high sugar content.

Your Schedule = Your Shopping List

So now that you've cleaned out your pantry and have a total mastery of what all the packaging means, what's next? Buying good food and ingredients! But I want you to try a new approach to thinking about what you buy. When it comes to the items for which you actually *need* to go grocery shopping, making a list is going to get you only so far. In fact, I'd argue that it can actually be quite *pointless* to make a list if you're not thinking about the whens of your food shopping as much as you're thinking about the whats.

Your work and activity *schedule* should provide the entire framework of your shopping list for any given week. Preplanning will help you avoid the following scenarios:

- I can't use any of this food I just bought because I have work dinners every night this week.

- I have no healthy food to eat at home.
- I have nothing to eat for breakfast/I have nothing to eat for snacks.
- I'm dying for a take-out pizza right now, and since I don't really have anything like it at home . . . welp, I'm picking one up when I leave work.
- Why don't I have anything here that I can take *with* me to eat on the run?

#protips

Before an item goes into your cart, consider these three questions, and adjust based on the recipe or meal you're looking to make by choosing said food or ingredient:

1. **Easy:** Does this make it easier for me to get meals on the table?
2. **Transparent:** Does the ingredients list on this product accurately reflect the marketing claims made on its packaging?
3. **Affordable:** Is this within my budget? Is there a less-expensive generic or store label item available that I could buy?

Assess Your Calendar

Before making your list or heading to the store, start with a hard analysis of your calendar. Here are some good questions you can use as prompts to help inform your shopping list as it relates to your schedule:

- How many nights are you eating at home? How many people will be at each meal?
- Where will you have breakfast and lunch each day? At home (if at home, how many people will be eating)? At the office? Out at a restaurant? On the go?

Figure out a menu for the meals you'll be eating at home. Obviously, the items that appear on your shopping list should be the ingredients for those meals; don't forget the snack items to keep up your schedule of eating every three to four hours.

Next: Make yourself a little chart with the following headings.

Stuff I'd Eat Mostly Every Day:	Stuff I'd Eat Mostly Every Week:	Stuff I Need In My Home to Make The Stuff I Eat Every Day And Every Week:

This is like a diagnostic tool for your own schedule based on *food*. (Seriously, you just have to do this *one time*—it's beyond illuminating!)

What Should This List Actually Look Like, Though?!

You're reading this book for a reason: You want to make a real, long-lasting change to your health and diet through the foods you eat. Here are a few tips regarding what should be in your cart.

Veggies: Start with fresh veggies to use in salads, soups, omelets, and sautés. Since ingredient prep is a major barrier to getting in those good-for-you foods (who wants to chop veggies after back-to-back meetings?!), buying prepared ingredients can be an easy way to mitigate the urge to say, *Whatever, I'm getting cheese fries,* and order takeout. Frozen vegetables, premade slaws, stir-fry veggie combos, or leafy blends are game changers when you're hoping to cut back on cooking time.

> When you get home from the store, wash, cut, and individually package your ingredients so that it's super easy to grab a day's servings as you're running out the door in the morning. And store these where you can visually see them in the fridge—not hidden behind your leftovers!

Fruit: Same deal. Use these as the base of most of your snacks, plus breakfast fruit that you'd want to add to yogurt, cereal, or smoothies.

Fun ways to turn fruit into speedy snacks: cubes of pineapple and clementine slices; bananas mixed with halved strawberries; or mango with blueberries—all of these are easy to toss into a ziplock bag with nuts or seeds and grab for your midday or mid-morning snack as you're running out the door.

Dairy: Hard-boiled eggs in bulk for snacks or egg salad, or use 'em as protein to top veggies with rice for a quick dinner. Low-fat, plain Greek yogurt or cottage cheese for dips or as a part of breakfast, and part-skim string cheese for toppings and snacks or as an ingredient in salads and sandwiches.

EGG LABELS, DECODED

Egg Carton Claims—What They *Really* Mean

Pasture-raised: These chickens roam on open grass, which allows them to both forage for food and eat supplemental feed. These typically cost more than other eggs because of the more expensive farming practices.

Cage-free: These chickens are not raised in cages, which gives them room to flap their wings. However, they often don't have access to sunlight.

Free-range: Think "cage-free" plus outdoor access, which makes these eggs a more affordable option than pasture-raised.

USDA organic: The only label that's federally regulated; organic farming practices ensure that these chickens are both free-range and cage-free. They're also fed 100 percent organic feed, meaning that all ingredients must also meet USDA standards.

Vegetarian-fed: These hens are fed mostly corn and soybeans. Look for omega-3s to be called out on the carton, meaning the feed's been enhanced with flaxseed or algae to optimize the nutrient profile (if you're even concerned), but all things considered, this claim bears no relationship to whether or not they're raised free-range or cage-free. In fact, all chicken feed is technically vegetarian, whether it's organic or not.

Gluten-free: This indicates that the chickens' feed is gluten-free, but this is a bit of a misleading claim. Gluten—even if it *was* in hen feed—wouldn't be present in the egg, since it's metabolized by a completely different pathway. This falls into the same category of unnecessary labeling and obvious marketing technique as potato chips being called cholesterol-free.

Add to Cart

☐ Produce of any kind—fresh or frozen, organic or conventionally grown
☐ Fruit canned in water or canned without syrup or any form of added sugar
☐ Canned vegetables and beans with "no salt added" (0 g) or "low sodium" (140 mg) or generally 230 mg of sodium per serving or less; no additional flavoring/ingredients other than preservatives (e.g., ascorbic acid; alpha-tocopherol)
☐ Unsweetened dried fruit and snacks; nuts, seeds, roasted bean-based snacks
☐ Unsweetened beverages, including caffeinated tea and coffee, seltzer/club soda, cow's milk and unsweetened plant-based milks
☐ Fish (canned, frozen, wild-caught Alaska salmon and tuna; sustainably farmed Norwegian salmon; fish sold at specialty retailers and mass-market retailers who are able to demonstrate traceability/origin of product)
☐ Whole, plant-based protein sources

100 percent whole grains: breads, English muffins, cereals.

Nuts and nut butters: Almonds, cashews, peanuts, pistachios, walnuts, and the ilk, depending on your personal taste and preference.

Pulses: All beans, peas, and lentils.

Seafood: Tuna, salmon, shrimp, sardines, anchovies, scallops, halibut, cod…you name it, ~~you should~~ I'd love for you to eat more of it. Canned, fresh, or frozen, there's lots of ways to enjoy seafood.

Meat and poultry: Lean cuts of beef; ground turkey or chicken; skinless turkey or chicken breasts.

Treats: Consciously indulging is a key component of better health. (More on that in chapter 7.)

Cooking oils: Olive oil, corn oil, canola oil, peanut oil, walnut oil, pecan oil, avocado oil, hemp seed oil—you don't need all of these, but you see where I'm going on this one: There are lots of options. Also an option? Butter. Yes, *butter*. (*In a book that says "diet" on the cover, no less!*) You need cooking oils and butter to make things you actually like to eat taste good, and you need to learn how to use these things without being afraid of them. We'll get to that in chapter 8.

Broth and stock: Low-sodium beef, chicken, and vegetable broths and stocks are handy for adding flavor to a multitude of dishes without adding unwanted fat or calories.

Condiments: Look for low-sodium versions of the usuals, including mustard, ketchup, soy sauce, and hot sauce; don't forget about hummus, guacamole, nut butters, and salsa.

Spices: Some spice staples to keep on hand: cayenne pepper, garlic and onion powders, turmeric, cinnamon, ginger, cumin, oregano, thyme, and rosemary.

Toppings for yogurt and fruit: Trail mixes, nut blends, chia/flax/hemp seeds—all of these have health benefits.

Caution!

- **Sugary beverages,** including juice (100 percent juice, "no sugar added" juice, etc.), sweetened coffee and tea, coffee creamers, smoothie drinks, and sodas.
- **Other products in which sugar—by any name—is the first ingredient,** for example, brown rice syrup, organic cane syrup/organic cane sugar, tapioca syrup, honey, agave, fruit juice puree, fruit puree, maple syrup, and caramel syrup.
- Products that show a **"protein isolate"** or **"protein blend"** as the first ingredient, which is commonly the case in energy bars.
- Products that state **"may contain hydrogenated/partially hydrogenated oils"** in the ingredients list.
- Products that identify with a particular fad diet as denoted on packaging (e.g., **"clean ingredients"**; **"Paleo"**).

❑ Breakfast/packaged foods with **nutrient marketing claims that are enticingly skewed toward school-aged interests (***marketing to kids = not so cool!***)** (e.g., sugar-sweetened breakfast cereal).

❑ Products that say **"naturally sweetened," "no sugar added," "no high-fructose corn syrup," "no artificial ingredients," "no artificial sweeteners,"** and use **"simple"** or **"simply"** in the product name or brand title while containing other forms of sweeteners, sodium, saturated fat, and emulsifiers.

Seafood Myths, Busted

Only 50 percent of women of childbearing age eat enough fish for proper fetal brain development should they become pregnant. Let's bust the top five myths on the superfood you're not getting enough of—and talk about how to get it back on your menu!

Seafood is hard to cook. False. It's one of the only foods that can truly go from freezer to table in minutes. And frozen shellfish—like shrimp and scallops—can stay in the freezer for up to six months when packaged properly. Ready-to-eat snack packs (like those from Bumble Bee and StarKist) are also handy for a good-for-you, omega-3-filled desk lunch or lunch on the go—you can add them to salad greens, sandwiches, or even whole-grain pasta.

Buying good seafood is expensive. Actually, it can be one of the most affordable proteins on the market! Plus, since it's deliciously satisfying, buying high-quality fish from your local retailer is cost-effective, as you need less than you think to serve the whole family: 4 ounces cooked with lots of veggies and 100 percent whole grains will provide a wholesome dinner for the whole family.

You should buy only "organic" fish. If you see markups on any seafood labeled "organic," run the other way. There's no such thing as organic fish—aquaculture isn't overseen by the USDA (which is the only way anything can be legally labeled "USDA organic"). Farm-raised is A-OK. Responsible farming practices include a zero-tolerance policy for water pollution, antibiotics, and parasiticides, and they employ sustainability practices verified by a third party. (This mimics the USDA organic "third-party" verification format for meat, but it's done without the federal government getting involved.) Anyone who is selling farmed fish at the fish counter should be able to provide the supermarket's policy and protocol on aquaculture practices, so you can (and should!) always ask if you're concerned. The best farm-raised and wild-caught fish, however, is typically sold at retailers who buy only from suppliers with strict processing and handling standards. Another interesting option is packaged seafood with verifiable UPC codes that you can type into a search engine on the company's website to find out exactly where your fish came from.

Compromise at the Supermarket = Self-Care

The fact that you've ditched your college ramen noodles and tossed the leftover Halloween candy doesn't mean you're doomed to tasteless food you won't enjoy eating. The idea is to purchase foods that you'll eat, enjoy, and feel satisfied by, but not foods that you'll be tempted to binge on for the sugar, salt, and fat. I've seen this compromise become a game changer for people of all shapes and sizes and with all types of different eating habits. We'll discuss it more in chapters to come, but for your grocery-shopping purposes, think about it this way: If you live for the taste of Nutella, I'm not going to ask you to quit enjoying a chocolaty, nutty treat—instead, look for something that has the same components but isn't quite as binge-able. For instance, chocolate hazelnut butter, which contains about 9 grams of sugar in the 2-tablespoon serving size, is super satisfying. This way, you optimize satiety without sacrificing flavor—a win for taste and health benefits. See page 106 for some other specific ideas on satisfying swaps.

CHEAT SHEET: PERSONAL SHOPPING GUIDELINES/ GOALS (AKA YOUR POCKET RD)

❑ **Snack bars:** 250 calories or less; >4 g fiber; >4 g protein; <6 g added sugar (as applicable, based on ingredients list)

> First ingredient must be a whole-food source other than sugar (by any name). Whole foods include: 100 percent whole grains, nuts or seeds, or fruit or vegetables, pulses.
> If the product contains fruit:
> *Potential bonus:* More than 4 g of protein with lower fiber content; more than 4 g of fiber with lower protein content.
> *Be wary of:* Claims of perceived health benefits, such as "vegan," "macrobiotic," "gluten-free," or "raw."

❑ **Crunchy snacks (vegetable- or grain-based chips, crackers, popcorn, pulse snacks):** 150 to 250 calories per serving; >3 g each of protein and fiber per serving; <6 g added sugar per serving; crackers should be <2 g sugar per serving and <2 g saturated fat per serving (up to 3 g if cheese-flavored/using real cheese); <230 mg sodium per serving (unless the product contains cheese; still must be under 300 mg)

> *Potential bonus:* More than 4 g of protein with lower fiber content; more than 4 g of fiber with lower protein content.
> *Be wary of:* Snack products that boast "superfood" qualities.

❑ **Bread:** 100 percent whole grain is the first ingredient; 120 calories or less per slice; ≤160 mg sodium per serving; ≥3 g fiber; >3 g protein; <3 g sugar

> *Potential bonus:* Higher fiber and/or protein content but with higher sugar content (allow no more than 3 g for a standard 28 g slice).

Be wary of: Claims such as "made with whole grains" or "whole grain" if 100 percent whole wheat or alternate grain flour is not the first ingredient.

❑ **Frozen breakfast and griddle cakes (2 waffles/pancakes/French toast slices):** 100 percent whole grain is the first ingredient; 200 calories or less per serving; >3 g fiber; <1 g saturated fat; <360 mg sodium
❑ **English muffin/bagel/sandwich thins:** 100 percent whole grain is the first ingredient; 180 to 220 calories; <230 mg sodium per serving; >3 g fiber; >3 g protein
❑ **Hot cereal (per 45 g standard serving size of instant packets or cups):** 100 percent whole grain or whole-grain blend is the first ingredient; >3 g fiber per serving; <5 g sugar per serving (unsweetened); <9 g sugar per serving (sweetened)

   Bonus: No added sugars/sweeteners (0 g/serving).

❑ **Cold cereal (per 1 cup):** 100 percent whole grain or whole-grain blend is the first ingredient; ≥5 g fiber per serving; ≥4 g protein per serving; ≤9 g sugar per serving (limit: 10 g sugar per 1-cup serving); ≤200 mg sodium

   Bonus: No added sugars/sweeteners (0 g/serving).

❑ **Granola (per ⅓- to ½-cup serving):** 200 to 250 calories; <6 g sugar; ≥3 g fiber; ≤2 g saturated fat; ≤200 mg sodium
❑ **Frozen muffins (per serving):** 100 percent whole grain, vegetable, or fruit must be the first ingredient; 150 calories; ≤10 g sugar; ≥3 g fiber; <300 mg sodium
❑ **Egg sandwiches/burritos/wraps/flatbreads:** 300 calories or less; ≥3 g fiber; ≥8 g protein; ≤480 mg sodium
❑ **Frozen entrées (no eggs):** 400 calories or less; ≥3 g fiber; ≥8 g protein; ≤480 mg sodium
❑ **Yogurt (4.4 ounces for whole milk; 5.3 ounces for 2% or skim):** 150 calories or less; ≤12 g sugar; ≥9 g protein

- ❏ **Cottage cheese (per ½-cup serving):** 90 calories or less; $\leq$280 mg sodium; if **sweetened with fruit:** $\leq$12 g sugar per 5.3-ounce container
- ❏ **Packaged cheese (per 1-ounce/28-gram serving):** 100 calories or less; $\leq$200 mg sodium; $\geq$6 g protein

  Bonus: Single-serving sizes.

- ❏ **Plain nut butters (per 2-tablespoon serving):** Only ingredients are "dry, roasted or raw nuts, or dry, roasted or raw nuts and salt"; 180 to 200 calories; 0 g sugar; $\leq$2.5 g saturated fat; $\geq$6 g protein; $\geq$3 g fiber
- ❏ **Flavored nut butters, seed butters, savory bean dips (per 2-tablespoon serving):** First ingredient is dry, roasted, or raw nut or seed; if oil is included: no hydrogenated oils, emulsifiers, or stabilizers (e.g., maltodextrin, hydrogenated vegetable oil); 180 to 200 calories; $\leq$4 g sugar; $\leq$2.51 g saturated fat; $\geq$6 g protein; $\geq$3 g fiber; $\leq$200 mg sodium
- ❏ **Sauces, condiments, and jams/jellies:** No sugar added to the product as per the *ingredients list* (cannot claim "no sugar added" but show a fruit or vegetable juice, puree, or juice concentrate used as sweetener); <230 mg sodium per ¼-cup serving in sauces/condiments; $\leq$6 g sugar in jams/jellies; $\leq$1 g saturated fat per serving in all condiments
- ❏ **Salad dressings:** Heart-healthy oil is the first ingredient (olive, avocado, etc.); $\leq$2 g saturated fat; $\leq$140 mg sodium; $\leq$2 g sugar
- ❏ **Beverages:** No sugar added to the beverage as per the *ingredients list* (exception is kombucha, in which sugar is essential to the fermentation process); nutrition facts are listed for entire bottle/box/pouch
- ❏ **Take-out/fast-food menu items:** 500 calories or less; $\leq$5 g saturated fat; $\leq$700 mg sodium per meal; $\leq$9 g added sugar. Red and processed meats at fast-food establishments are excluded.
- ❏ **Trail mixes/nuts/seeds:** Dry roasted or raw nuts/seeds; if it contains dried fruit, there is no sugar added; <140 mg sodium per serving

  Bonus: Single-serving sizes available.

❑ **Spices/seasoning:** <140 mg sodium per serving
❑ **Veggie burgers/vegetarian meat replacements:** First ingredient is a whole food (e.g., vegetables, beans, whole grains, sweet potatoes); ≤2.5 g saturated fat; ≤300 mg sodium
❑ **Soup (can or tetra-pack):** <600 mg sodium (25% RDI) if the soup provides one or more servings of vegetables; ≤460 mg sodium (20% RDI) if the soup provides 0 servings of vegetables

7

Everyone Says I Have to Cut Back on Sugar to Lose Weight, but There's Sugar in Everything!

By the end of this chapter, you will…

- understand that sugar addiction is "fake news" and how we got there;
- know the difference between naturally occurring and added sugars;
- be able to read any food label and determine if it contains added sugar;
- know how to spot a sneaky sugar pseudonym;
- kick stupid sugar to the curb so that you can eat sweets you love; and
- eat dessert every day (seriously).

First, Let's Talk About Dessert

Sugar gets a bad rap because it's everywhere. A 2014 study from the *American Journal of Clinical Nutrition* revealed the sources of most of the added sugars Americans consume: 34.4 percent from sugary soda and sports drinks; 12.7 percent from grain-based desserts (e.g., baked goods); 8 percent from fruit drinks (e.g., juice and juice cousins, such as lemonade, etc.); 6.7 percent from candy; and 5.6 percent from dairy desserts (e.g., ice cream). And where do we usually buy these sneaky sugar sources? Wherever we shop: 65 to 76 percent of added sugars come from grocery or supermarket shelves. Another study from the *British Journal of Medicine* (2016) using National Health and Nutrition Examination Surveys data revealed something along the same lines: About 60 percent of our total calorie intake and 90 percent of our intake of added sugars come from ultraprocessed foods.

What we can learn from these studies, which draw on epidemiological data to show us what we're *currently* eating in the name of informing us how to make better choices for the future? The supermarket, gas station, quick-mart, local grocer, and corner deli are where we buy most of our added sugar, and we're buying it in the forms of bottled drinks and packaged foods—*not* straight sugar cubes or treats we've made for ourselves at home.

Fun little fact: When you see "4 g sugar" on a label, that equals *1 teaspoon* of sugar. If you start thinking about grams of sugar in baking measurements, it's easier to get your mind around where you'd like to add more and where you'd prefer to cut back.

This list shows the amount of sugar contained in some common foods:

- One 12-ounce regular soda: 26 g (6.5 teaspoons)
- One whole bag of peanut M&M's: 25 g (6.25 teaspoons)
- One ½ cup of ice cream: 22 to 32 g, depending on flavor (5.5 to 8 teaspoons)
- One 16-ounce chai tea latte: 42 g (10.5 teaspoons)
- One Blow Pop: 15 g (3.75 teaspoons)
- One frozen margarita: 65 g (16.25 teaspoons)
- One 2-tablespoon serving of ketchup: 8 g (2 teaspoons)
- Nine Hershey's Kisses: 26 g (6.5 teaspoons)
- One 12-ounce Starbucks "Refresher": 26 g (6.5 teaspoons)
- One San Pellegrino (plain or any flavor): 0 g

How Much Sugar Should You Eat?

The American Heart Association says that men should aim to limit added sugar to 9 teaspoons per day (36 g), and women should aim for 6 teaspoons per day (24 g). A slightly more liberal recommendation comes from the USDA/HHS: The *Dietary Guidelines for Americans* recommends that we limit added sugar to 10 percent per day, which you'll see on the new FDA food label using 200 calories (10 percent of a 2,000-calorie diet), expressed as percent daily value. The World Health Organization makes a similar statement, sans calorie definition: "Limit added sugars to 10% of total calories per day."

That will give you a head start, but the most important weapon you have against eating too much sugar is label reading. When you're making your choice of a sweet treat or a dessert, compare the Nutrition Facts labels and ingredients lists to make the most nutritious choice. If you take a minute to just think through (or even better: Write it down!) what types of foods you normally eat that might have added sugar—ones you think might be ever-so-slightly susceptible to the infiltration of sugar for the purpose of taste or preservation, or in any sweetened beverage form of any kind—you may find a whole bunch of sneaky places that sugar hides out in order to contribute to your whole day. So, if we think about it more in the context of what you'd rather have—a pre-sweetened iced tea, or a bag of previously off-limits candy or cookie, or a postdinner frozen dessert, or a chocolate bar—doesn't the choice seem exceptionally easy? It is. Why have juice when you could *eat vegetables* and actually enjoy your dessert, too?!

Sugar "Addiction": The Mother of All Diet Myths

In recent years, there have been a slew of books, documentaries, articles, and research reports that delve into sugar metabolism and "expose" the various "dangers" of eating sugar. Some, like the documentary *Fed Up* (2014), liken sugar to a poison that leads to childhood obesity. Others, such as CBS's *60 Minutes* story "Sugar" (2012) and BBC's documentary *The Truth About Sugar* (2015) have likened our bodies' response to sugar as "toxic"—"addictive" in the same way one might become addicted to narcotics. (All of these have at least *some* cogent, evidence-based info in there!) On top of all this, we still see and read the constant battle in the media between epidemiologists and physicians regarding the "low-carb" versus "low-fat" controversy, leaving us even more confused. Here's what I've heard this confusion *sound like* among colleagues, friends, and lots of strangers:

- "Well, we used to think that carbs were good for us—now we know better!"
- "Carbs are sugar, and the *DGA* wants us to eat six servings a day?! That's ridiculous!"

- "Sugar is addictive."
- "Have you considered taking [insert prescription medication here] to help you with your sugar addiction? Let me write you a script."
- "It's okay to eat grains, but it's not okay to eat sugar."
- "Cut back on sugar—and don't forget, fruit is high in sugar, too, you know."
- "I'm on this keto diet because sugar is killing us."
- "Cut out the candy, cookies, pies, cakes, baked goods—you know, *all that sugar* you're eating."
- "If you don't cut back on sugar, you're at a higher risk for diabetes."

It's this type of thinking and these types of statements that lead us right back to demoralization via diet culture. We're not victims of food, nor are we lab rats; we are human beings with thoughts, feelings, ideas, and *real lives* that involve eating more than one nutrient in isolation!

In research, scientists often look specifically at a neurological pathway that identifies a "trigger" in a sweet taste (food) that is responsible for the feeling of receiving a happy reward (the feeling we get from serotonin). But looking at the "treat and reward" neuronal pathway is only one piece of the biochemistry puzzle, and it doesn't consider what *else* is happening in your body when you're eating sugar—and, therefore, *why* the timing and the type of treat you're eating are critical for maximizing that treat-and-reward pathway to begin with.

Bottom line: *You* are in control. How physically full you *feel while you eat* is directly related to everything else you're eating at one meal, in an hour, in a day, or tomorrow. So saying that we are capable of being addicted to sugar falls short of acknowledging what humans actually are—people who eat a wide variety of meals of mixed nutrients, with mixed nutritional value!

Registered dietitians are trained to look at your whole clinical picture when reviewing your nutrition-related needs. Isolating a neuronal pathway that is *similar* to that of addiction is *not* accounting for the everyday factors of your personal lifestyle—where you eat, when you eat, and why you eat sugar! Are you eating candy on an empty stomach, or are you eating a piece of it after a meal? Are you drinking sugar without realizing it? Are you eating tons of sugar because you had absolutely no idea it was in nearly everything you have in your fridge/pantry/freezer at the moment? Are you eating sugar out of boredom? Sadness? Or maybe you realized after reading the first half of this book that actually, you're not "out of control" or "eating your feelings" *at all* around sugar—in fact, you feel out of control around sugar because you have a tendency to *start sh*t with your demons* because you didn't have enough at breakfast, didn't drink enough water, skipped a snack today, and had a pretty unsatisfying meal (read: pasta sans protein; chicken sans carb) and now you're up late finishing work and all you can think about is licorice. These are a few of the many, often unmindful ways that sugar comes into our foods and our lives. Implying that the foods we eat are so powerful over us that we have no control or say in what or when we eat is demoralizing, as noted above. Besides all of this, it ignores a huge fact: This is one "addiction" that we can cure with a little education, mindfulness, and staying conscientious about our food choices.

The Three T's of Sweets: Real Treats, No Tricks

Back in chapter 2, we talked about the three T's as a means to avoid skipping meals. They are **timing**—eating every three to four hours; **type**—always eating a combination of foods that are nutrient-dense; and **tools**—making sure you have a ready list of go-to places and handy access to food sources that will allow you to make healthful food choices.

Now we're going to take the concept of the three T's—timing, type, and tools—and adapt it, with different guidelines, to make daily dessert work for you.

Timing of treats: I *rarely* say "never," but in the context of dessert, I'd urge you to think about the following before you dive in for a treat you actually like and want to eat regularly:

a. **Keep sugars camouflaged in "healthy" costumes *away* from your breakfast meal.** Eating an all-carb breakfast is deadly for your energy and sets you up for a downward spiral throughout the day. Depending on who you are, this may or may not have affected you before, or it may be affecting you without your realizing it. So while I'd never say "no candy for breakfast" (who are we kidding—sometimes we all need to put peanuts and chocolate together and call it breakfast when we're in a bind!), I will say "no high-sugar foods masquerading as 'healthy' for breakfast," because you need to make sure your breakfast is a combo of protein, fat, and fiber, which will give you sustained energy—not the blood sugar spike and crash that come with things such as a bagel, a donut, a gluten-free donut, a breakfast pastry, a gluten-free breakfast pastry, a bottled juice beverage, a store-bought smoothie, a sweetened cereal or oatmeal, a sweetened yogurt or yogurt drink, and plant-based milks that are "plain" but not "unsweetened." By avoiding sneaky sugar traps at breakfast, you're starting your day off on a more conscious, more energized foot that helps you to stay satisfied throughout the morning and up until lunch, and also puts you in the mind-set of "I'm in the driver's seat—I'll decide when I want to eat sugar!" (Right?!)

b. **Consider when to eat treats based on your schedule:** Here's the deal—if you're a type 1 diabetic, you already know this by now. But for some, it may come as a surprise that your body needs fifteen minutes to digest and absorb about 15 grams of carbs from sugar (or carbs in their simplest biochemical form). This time can vary depending on the type of food you eat, but a similar process occurs regardless. So you eat some sugar; your body needs fifteen minutes to get that through your GI tract and into your bloodstream to raise your sugar level; and from there, you've got about another fifteen minutes to really use that sugar for something (*ride that blood sugar high!*) or to experience a crash (*a quick descent into exhaustion*) from that. Think about what you'll be doing in the next half hour before you go hard on the jelly beans, soda, juice, fro-yo, and the ilk. That's why it's usually my #protip to recommend eating dessert in the evening, when it's *encouraged* for you to come down from that high and sleep like a baby. Even better: Sometimes a little treat fifteen minutes before getting into bed can even *help* cut the sheep-counting out of the equation and help knock you right into a REM cycle! (Finicky sleepers: Proceed with caution.)

Type of sugar-containing food: The *quality* of your treat or dessert often matters more than the *quantity*, but what that actually means in real life is personal to you. For example, maybe you live for Raisinets (*in which case please don't bring them anywhere near me, thanks!*). And sure, there are some types of treats that are better than others, but the reasons why have to do with satiety and personal preferences, not purely the Nutrition Facts label, grams of sugar, or calorie count. So with that in mind, it's got to be something you actually enjoy—you want to make the choice to drink a cold-pressed coconut something as your dessert? *Do you?!* The reason it's called a treat and not "lunch" is that it's not comprising 100 percent of everything you eat, all day, every day. If you're reading this and shaking your head, saying, *"No! I love sugar! I want to bathe in sugar and eat it in everything!"* listen up: One of the biggest trends I've noticed among clients is that many assume they have a personal "problem" with sugar, when actually, they're doing one of three things:

- Consuming excess sugar from unlikely food sources of it, without *knowing* that those foods contain sugar, in forms that easily add up quickly (condiments, sauces, bread products, cereals, crackers, chips, milks, yogurts, protein bars, protein shakes, juices, supplements, and powders).

- Attempting to Band-Aid a love of sugar with items that are just not going to cut it (like a banana when they want a donut) and subsequently eating *way* more than they need over the course of a day as a result of "avoiding sugar."

- Not following their Right-Now Rules (eat breakfast every day, eat every three to four hours, stay accountable) and *not* being aware of their willpower sh*t starters (not drinking enough water, not getting enough sleep, and having an irregular exercise/physical activity schedule).

That's why quality is the emphasis here. For most of us, sugar adds up in our diets in ways that have much more to do with our lifestyle than they do with our making a conscious decision to have something sweet.

My goal is to empower you to make a choice about when you want to eat sugar . . . which is why I frame a lot of this information in the context of "dessert" (*because, that's what sugar's initial intended role in our food supply once was, Paula!*). It's all designed to empower you to *choose* your sweets in the context of your everyday lifestyle, not to be pigeonholed into thinking that sugar is "killing you" or "making you fat."

Tools: Your main tools for more conscientiously choosing sugar-containing treats or desserts are nutrition knowledge and label reading. Let's revisit label reading now.

Label Reading 101: First, Determine a "Guesstimate" of Naturally Occurring Sugars and the Amount of Added Sugars

Quick recap: There are two types of sugars in foods and beverages: naturally occurring and added.

Naturally occurring sugars, sugars that are naturally found in foods, include **fructose** (fruit sugar), which is found in—you guessed it—fruit, honey, and root veggies; **lactose** (milk sugar), which is found in dairy products; and **sucrose** (a combo of glucose and fructose), which is found naturally in carbohydrates of all types, including all types of produce.

Added sugars are sugars, syrups, fruit juice concentrates, and caloric sweeteners that are added to foods or beverages during their preparation or processing.

Here are some categories of carb-based foods that often contain added sugars for flavor and preservation:

- Sweetened grain-based products
- Sweetened dairy products and non-dairy alternatives
- Sweetened foods and drinks with veggies or fruit as the base
- Condiments, toppings, syrups, and soft drinks

So now you know the difference between naturally occurring sugars and added sugars, and you have a pretty good idea of which foods contain them. Sounds simple, right?

Well, it's a *teensy* bit more *nebulous* than that.

What makes this a little more complicated is that fruit contains about 15 grams of naturally occurring fructose sugar per unit of small, whole fruit (e.g., one small apple, orange, or teensy banana) or a serving of a cup of fruit (e.g., grapes). Similarly, a dairy product is going to have about 12 grams of sugar per 8-ounce cup of milk. This means that when you're at the supermarket checking for added sugar on food labels, you might get a little thrown off by the fact that (a) sugar has *lots* of aliases (we'll get to that in a minute), and (b) it's hard to tell whether there's naturally occurring sugar *and* added sugar in a product. The new labels will make life easier, but until *everyone* boards that train in 2021, let's simplify this process by checking out a few ways labels can be confusing and how to get an estimate on the added sugar content of each.

Fage 2% 7-ounce cup	Fage 2% Cherry split cup
140 calories	120 calories
4 g fat	2.5 g fat
2.5 g saturated fat	1.5 g saturated fat
65 mg sodium	40 mg sodium
6 g total carbs	13 g total carbs
6 g sugar	11 g sugar
20 g protein	12 g protein

(Adapted from Fage website, www.fageusa.com, accessed June 2018)

The left side is the plain version of a 2% yogurt; the right side is a sweetened version. In a 7-ounce (about ⅔ cup) container of plain yogurt, you've got 6 grams of naturally occurring lactose. The product isn't sweetened, which you know by looking at the ingredients list, right? No sugary ingredients—just milk, cream, and live and active cultures (*five* is your golden number to ensure you're buying something with a solid smattering of beneficial bacteria for your GI tract—you'll recognize these by their regal-sounding Latin names, like *Bacillus coagulans*). The right side shows that on top of the amount of naturally occurring lactose in the product, manufacturers would have had to add sugar to this split cup in order to make that cherry deliciousness that comes along with it. Since the amount of yogurt you actually get in a split cup (or any "fruit at the bottom" or "blended" type of yogurt) is *less* than a plain version by nature of the smaller-sized split cup and food processing, we can't *just* say there's "5 grams added sugar" (sugars = 11 g; subtract the 6 you know is in the plain version, and you get 5 g of added sugar by this estimation). But we *can* use that information to provide us with a rough estimate. Using this example, that would mean that the amount of added sugar in a sweetened version is roughly 1.5 tablespoons (*likely a little* more, *but let's be generous because minutia is a joy killer, Phyllis! You're still eating a wholesome, protein-packed, real food!*).

This example shows you how naturally occurring sugars and added sugars can coexist in the same product and be both a nutritious choice *and* a more indulgent choice—depending on your preferences and how you're incorporating this type of snack into your day. My advice would be to buy the plain version, not because I'm a monster who hates cherries (I love them, in fact!) but because you get more bang for your buck when you buy plain: *More yogurt!* If I buy the version on the left, I can add my own fruit, or I could add literal sugar if I felt so inclined (though I'd opt for more whole fruit, since it's got tons o' fiber...hint, hint). But I can *also* use it in savory foods, too—a dip! A high-protein sour cream swap! In a smoothie! With my breakfast! And my lunch! And my *dinner! OMG I can even use this to make dessert!*

(*Does it do dishes?*)

At the end of the day, you can't make informed decisions if you don't have the information to begin with. Information gives you options, and options give you freedom within a clearly defined framework to make choices that empower you and meet *your* personal needs.

Let's use another example with fruit.

"Plain" Applesauce

90 calories, 0g fat, 0 mg sodium, 24 g carbohydrates, 1 g fiber, 22 g sugar, 0 g protein, 20% DV vitamin C, 2% potassium

Ingredients

Apples, high-fructose corn syrup, water, ascorbic acid (vitamin C)

(Adapted from Mott's website, www.motts.com, accessed June 2018)

Plain, Unsweetened Applesauce

50 calories, 0 g fat, 0 mg sodium, 13 g total carbohydrates; 1 g fiber, 11 g sugar, 0 g protein, 20% DV vitamin C, 2% DV potassium

Ingredients

Apples, water, ascorbic acid (vitamin C)

(Adapted from Mott's website, www.motts.com, accessed June 2018)

One Apple

80 calories, 0 g saturated fat, 0 mg cholesterol, 1 mg sodium, 159 mg potassium, 21 g carbohydrates, 4 g fiber, 15 g sugar, <1 g protein, 11% DV vitamin C

(Source: USDA Nutrient Analysis Library, "Apple Nutrition Facts," accessed June 2018)

If one small apple is about 15 grams of naturally occurring sugar, unsweetened applesauce is 11 grams of naturally occurring sugar, because you're getting less than one apple in that small little pouch. But the sweetened applesauce takes the 11–15 grams of naturally occurring sugar that you'd eat in an unsweetened version or a whole apple, and *adds 7 grams* of sugar compared to an apple, and *11 grams* of sugar if you're comparing it to an unsweetened version. That's about 2–3 teaspoons of added sugar per serving! Your other tip-off? There's high-fructose corn syrup in the sweet type, which indicates that the product itself is sweet, despite the fact that it's considered "plain" because the brand makes *other flavors of applesauce*—like cinnamon and "tropical."

So which one do you pick? Personally, I'd urge you to skip the sweetened applesauce, because I think it's a throwaway of 2–3 teaspoons of sugar that didn't really fill you up—neither type of applesauce has much by way of actual fiber (about 1 g), while the apple has about 4 grams of fiber (and often can pack up to 6 g, depending on the type). Applesauce aficionados? Go for it! But if you love fruit in fruit form and treats in dessert form, go for the apple to get the most nutritional benefit (water, fiber, and anti-oxidants that can't possibly be processed away since you're eating a whole fruit).

Is It True That Fat-Free Milk Has More Sugar Than Whole Milk?

Nope. Because of the way milk is processed, there will be a higher percentage of calories coming from naturally occurring sugar that was already present in the milk when it first left the udder. To make skim (nonfat) milk, the fat has to be removed, meaning that the product's remaining calories will be from lactose sugar and animal protein, leading those to—*of course*—be the predominant source of calories in the milk that remains after dairy-fat elimination *happened*. But no matter what type of cow's milk you choose, you'll always see "12 g" total carbs, and 12 g of total sugar per serving. And similarly, you'll also always see 8 g of protein per serving. Why? Because the protein and carbs aren't removed—just the fat source. Milk goes from about 8 g fat to 0 g fat, and one serving goes from 150 calories per cup to about 80–90 calories per cup (depends on the brand—some are more like 100, and that's related to processing and filtration-system differences). Since fat is 9 calories per gram, and protein and carbs are each 4 calories per gram, the idea that there's any *added* sugar, that there's a *higher amount* of sugar, or that the product goes up in sugar simply because the fat was removed can really be answered with some simple math:

4 calories/g of carbohydrates × 12 g/1 cup = 48 calories from carbs; 4 calories/g of protein × 8 g/1 cup = 32. 48 + 32 = 80 calories per cup of nonfat milk.

> **Bottom line:** If you say that there's a higher percentage of calories coming from sugar in nonfat milk than in whole milk, you'd be 100 percent correct. But the nuance is distinct and important. It makes it sound like you'd said, "There's more sugar in nonfat milk!"—right? And that's 100 percent *wrong*.
>
> *(Unless, of course, it's a flavored milk…in which case, that's another can of worms.)*

Last on our list of examples to ~~exploit~~ discuss: grain-based products, which range from traditional desserts (such as cookies and cakes) to things like cereal, breakfast bars, and granola bars.

What makes these a little easier for sugar-spotting is that you don't have to consider naturally occurring sugar when you're thinking through a "what should I buy?" amidst the grains and flour of the grocery store. Why? Because it's all added! While carbs are digested and absorbed similarly, grains and other types of flour (e.g., corn) provide a negligible amount in naturally occurring form (hence why they're so ubiquitous at the supermarket) and used as a base for products sweet *or* savory in flavor.

This is a breakfast biscuit in the flavor of "Golden Oats."

Belvita Golden Oats Breakfast Biscuit

1 pack: 230 calories, 8 g total fat, 0.5 g saturated fat, 0 g trans fat, 0 mg cholesterol, 220 mg sodium, 85% daily value potassium, 35 g total carbohydrates, 3 g fiber, 11 g sugar, 4 g protein

Ingredients

Whole-grain blend (rolled oats, rye flakes), enriched flour (wheat flour, niacin, reduced iron, thiamin mononitrate [vitamin B_1], riboflavin [vitamin B_2], folic acid), canola oil, sugar, whole-grain wheat flour, evaporated cane sugar, malt syrup (from corn and barley), invert sugar, baking soda, salt, soy lecithin, disodium pyrophosphate, DATEM, ferric orthophosphate

(continued)

(iron), niacinamide, pyridoxine hydrochloride (vitamin B$_6$), riboflavin (vitamin B$_2$), thiamin mononitrate (vitamin B$_1$).

Contains: wheat, soy.

(Adapted from Belvita Breakfast website, of Mondelez International, http://www.belvitabreakfast.com, accessed June 2018.)

KIND Snacks Honey Oat Breakfast Bar

220 calories, 8 g fat, 0.5 g saturated fat, 0 g trans fat, 9 mg cholesterol, 30 mg sodium, 33 g total carb, dietary fiber 5 g, 9 g sugar, 4 g protein

Ingredients

Whole-grain oats, sugar, canola oil, rice flour, honey, salt, brown sugar syrup, baking soda, soy lecithin, natural flavor.

(Adapted from KIND website, www.kindsnacks.com, accessed June 2018.)

See how both brands have a sugar value listed in their nutrition facts that is *lower* than the number of "total carbs"? When you're buying something made from grains, sugars are left blank or listed as "0 g sugar" when there's nothing sweet added to the product. It won't change the fact that the product has *carbohydrates* because it *is* mostly carbohydrates. But why do you see "9 g" listed under sugar for each type of granola/breakfast bar? Because there's about 3 teaspoons added to each product to make it a sweet and tasty little grain—instead of you eating a sensible slice of whole-grain bread or a 100 percent whole-grain oatmeal cup.

SUGAR SIRENS

Sugar sirens are words on packaging and food labels that are designed to turn you from a strong, fearless, highly prepared Unstoppable Ulysses traveling the Aegean to a very confused, overwhelmed, and Befuddled Belinda— who may or may not make some purchases at the grocery store, restaurant, or convenience store because she was swayed by sugar sirens—the claims made on sugar-containing packaging that boast about their lack of sugar content when in fact they've tapped into an FDA regulation labeling loophole that allows them to use said terms for the sake of distracting you/luring you/ convincing you to buy their product. Some great examples of this include:

No refined sugar!
Made with coconut sugar!
Low glycemic index!
Fat-free (on a bag of sour candy or jelly beans or Swedish fish)!
No high-fructose corn syrup!
Sweetened with agave nectar!
Made with organic cane sugar!
Clean sugar!
Raw sugar!
Natural!
Fair Trade Certified!

We've already reviewed the many reasons why these claims can be confusing, but when it comes to sneaky sugar, this is where we've really got to get serious about reading the fine print. It's so dang easy for all of us to fall victim to sugar sirens that sometimes we may "fall" for the claim "no high-fructose corn syrup!" even when there is regular CORN SYRUP listed as the second ingredient! Places you'll find this? Cereal, in particular, but it's also abundant in any baked good, breakfast pastry, or sugar-containing condiment.

Bottom line: You don't need to add sugar to things made *with or from a source of sugar.* Of course, this is a free country—you *can* if that's how you truly enjoy eating your sweets! But from my POV, if we got a little clearer with ourselves about where we could stand to skip out on the sugar, it would be a whole lot more fun to have an ice cream cone and call it a day, right?

Bottom line: If the first ingredient of a product is a sugar by *any name,* it's still sugar, which makes the product still *mostly dessert,* not a "health food" or a "snack." Again, the choice to determine what makes something dessert is yours, so I leave it to you to make that call—so long as you're choosing things because you like the flavor, not the marketing fluff.

Consider Letting Go of Sugary Beverages

A quick backstory on calorie-containing beverages for you history buffs out there. Diets high in sugar-containing (aka calorie-containing) beverages are linked to a higher risk of overweight/obese BMI, weight gain, and chronic disease risk versus diets with minimal sugar-containing-beverage intake. There's about a zillion studies that support this concept, and it's no surprise as to why. When you drink 200 calories worth of cola, you're unlikely to feel full because (a) no fiber, (b) no protein, and (c) no fat. The calories are coming from simple sugars, likely in the form of glucose, fructose, and sucrose, and they're quickly digested and absorbed in your GI tract because your mouth, esophagus, stomach, and intestines literally have to do *zero* work to digest and absorb these nutrients (passive diffusion, people!). Remember: In order to achieve not only *fullness* but also *satiety*, you'll need real, whole foods that are filled with water and fiber, plus protein and some good-for-you fat.

On the other hand, on your most exhausted, least hydrated, most hangry day ever, if you were to eat 200 calories worth of nuts, you would at *worst* feel as though you were still peckish, but on your way to filling up. At best, you'd feel totally sated and like you didn't need another snack until your next meal in three to four hours (because you follow directions like a boss).

Sugar Myth Busting

High-Fructose Corn Syrup Is Lethal, Though, Isn't It?

Nope, it's not. High-fructose corn syrup is made from corn, and sugar is made from sugarcane (both *plants*, but the former has more fructose than glucose, and vice versa in the latter). Fructose is metabolized *ever so slightly* differently from glucose, but the differences in their actual *food sources* have been completely *abused* by the info jungle (one-off study findings in the news, marketing campaigns, and research that's examined differences in human metabolism of these predominant types of simple sugar in each ingredient). But the bottom line is that regardless of the type of sweetener you're consuming: If you're overdoing it on *total grams of sucrose*, aka total grams of sugar from both or either type, you're at a higher risk for adverse health effects and weight gain. If you're not, then the nuances in metabolism and animal-model data differences that affect metabolism are basically *null and void*, right?! The problem with much of the data on this topic is that the studies are conducted through providing high doses of glucose or fructose and examining differences in metabolism, biochemistry, and fat distribution—but that's (a) only performed in animal studies, and (b) irrelevant, since that's not the way we consumers eat food to begin with. (*That cola is more than just corn syrup, Shelby!*). Ads and commercials touting the benefit of one versus the other? That's using a sliver of science to make for a smarter marketing campaign, my friends. (*And by now, you're better than that!*)

What About Juice and Smoothies? And What If I Made My Own?

Alright, kids, now let's get into the AP class of sugar. Here's the story with beverages: Not all of them actually have added sugar, or even have an FDA-approved version of added sugar. But since all of them that *have any kind of sugar at all* provide a blood sugar spike of those passively diffusing glucose molecules from your intestine into your bloodstream, they're all "counting" as sugary for the purpose of this book. I know, I know—this upsets you greatly. But let me explain for a moment: Sugar-containing beverages, by nature of what they are (sugar = 4 calories/gram) are *calorie-containing beverages*. And for the purposes of overall health, weight management and weight loss, sleeping better at night, and loving our lives just a teensy bit more: Beverages containing calories do not serve one of the main intended purposes of food to begin with, which is *to actually fill you up and make you feel satisfied by the food you eat!* And certainly, unless some of you are having milkshakes *daily*, you would likely be much more excited to learn that you could have some sparkling H_2O and dig in to dessert in place of having that same amount in liquid form, no?

Now, if you and your family are stuck on all sorts of sugary bevs and you love your holy-basil-and-broccolini "tonic" so much that you can't think about anything else and you're ready to throw this book into the blender simply because I called juice (and its cousins, tonic elixir, smoothie, fruit "water") a sugar-sweetened beverage, well—hold up: *I'm* grouping sugar-containing beverages—natural or otherwise—into the category of beverages containing sugar because these are still "counting" as calories that you're consuming—regardless of smart and clever marketing tactics, or the fact that they originally *came from produce*. They also "count" because of their direct impact on blood sugar: If you're delivering sugar to your cells in this concentrated form (fruit juice) and without a source of fiber (that's removed in the process), then you're spiking sugar without actually reaping the same satiety benefits you'd otherwise get from, say, a milkshake or a brownie (those both contain fat and some protein, which means they take longer to digest and absorb throughout your GI tract and therefore have a less immediate impact on your glycemic response to eating sweets).

To clarify: I'm assuming you *choose* to drink milkshakes or eat brownies once in a while, but the point is that you would, knowing that these are foods that are pretty up front about being what they are (treats!), make the choice to eat them knowing that they're desserts. By contrast, you may not have fully realized that kale-pineapple-hot-sauce-agave juice or some other sweet drink could contain the same amount of sugar, even though it's dressed up in a mason jar with health claims splashed across its packaging—right? Having this knowledge empowers you to make that choice, rather than consume something you thought was #clean #healthy #vegan but has the same amount of sugar from a more concentrated source—even though it's "all natural."

For context: One whole orange is about 60 calories and 15 grams sugar; one serving of juice (a measly ½ cup, or 4 ounces) about the same, so the choice (to juice or not to juice) is absolutely, 100 percent (naturally!) *yours* to make. Most of us, though (grown-ups *especially!*), aren't limiting ourselves to a shot glass worth of the sweet stuff, so just know that you're better off eating the *whole fruit*, not just the juice that fruit contains—regardless of processing technique, price point, packaging, or celebrity endorser.

BEHOLD, THE POWER OF CHEWING!

Making your own smoothies works, too, particularly when you're making them at home using plain, unsweetened Greek yogurt, any type of fruit or vegetable (or all of the fruits and vegetables!) you can find, and a tablespoon or two of nut butter; adding flavor from spices; and using ice for liquid (or an unsweetened plant-based milk or regular milk). But the reason I'm not the biggest proponent of the smoothie—homemade or otherwise—is because in practice, I simply have not found that my clients feel particularly *filled up* from drinking a smoothie as a meal—no matter *how many calories and grams of protein are in there!* For whatever reason, it just *feels* to most of us like it's a snack, not an "off to the races!" meal on which you can go for hours. Part of that is because when you don't actually *chew your food* (it's blended for you already!—your internal organs have to do less to get everything moving along) there's no further significant amount of digestion that takes place in your stomach. The intestine can get to work doing all of its absorptive business while you carry on living your life, dreaming about what time lunch is going to be today. Chewing brings a little bit more heavy lifting by the stomach and lower GI tract, provides you with a sensory experience from flavor, and increases mindfulness as you go—you bite, chew, think, meditate, namaste, swallow...you catch my drift.

Decide If This Item Is "Worth It" for You to Miss Dessert Today

If you think about the ability to eat dessert without worry, I'd encourage you to think about foods you like that *also have* added sugar in these terms:

1. Reference the numbers: fruit = 15 g sugar, and dairy = 12 g sugar. These are the naturally occurring sugars you'll find in a *full serving of fruit or dairy.* Use them as a jumping-off point if the product has either ingredient in there already.
2. Scan the label for added sugar—if it's 4 g, it's a teaspoon—and add up from there.
3. Read ingredients: The first ingredient should be a real, whole food—not sugar by a different alias, or sugar itself.
4. Question the value: Is this food worth me eating less dessert? Is it worth skipping dessert entirely? Which things should I choose "unsweetened" today if I go for this?
5. Eat. (Or don't eat.)

Eat Food, Not Food Claims

When it comes to added sugar, it does *not* matter whether the product is USDA organic, non-GMO project verified, fair trade certified, raw, refined, free of artificial colors, free of artificial flavors, gluten-free, dairy-free, vegan, paleo, Whole30 approved. That's why you've got to check the labels if you want to really *know* for sure what's in there. By relying on a claim or a health halo, you're basically just stepping on your own foot in terms of your health. So while something like a cereal product with berries in it can make a statement like "no added sugar" because it's using *freeze-dried berries*, it can also make a claim like "no artificial ingredients"—but are you really eating a fresh bowl of strawberries?! Nope.

I'm not out to throw shade on cereal or strawberries or sugar, to be clear. But I do think it's important that we don't let claims run our supermarket shopping (and therefore our wallets and our health) either. So with that in mind, keep these handy #protips in mind, which can serve as a reminder for you when you're searching for snacks:

- Anything that's linked to an agricultural statement (organic, natural, fair trade, non-GMO) is related to a production method and bears no relationship to actual nutritional content.
- Any claim pertaining to a nutrient or a food group other than sugar *or fat* bears no relationship to the nutritional content of the product. "Free from X" is a relatively new term that we are using left and right, so it may be difficult to recall (when you're piled under a myriad of potato chips and popcorn and salsa jars on aisle four) that the only nutrients that provide energy, aka calories, are carbohydrates, protein, and fat.
- The more processed the foods we try and trick ourselves into believing *are actually real*, the more confused we become. Fresh vegetables, fruit, 100 percent whole grains, lean protein sources (including eggs and low-fat dairy), plus nuts and seeds all contain vitamins, minerals, and other nutrients that fight chronic disease and prevent weight gain. Plus, we tend to feel more satisfied when we eat real, whole foods (especially those that are plant-based) because they're higher

in fiber and water content than others—meaning they help us feel fuller, longer.

I Can't Drink Diet Drinks Because That's Cyanide, Right?

Sure you can. Controversial, I know, but if your GI tract is A-OK with sugar substitutes, then you can use them—and you *should* use them if you love sugar-sweetened beverages and are otherwise living a life of chronic dehydration. (*How does your skin survive in winter?!*) Here's why there's confusion in this space: A clinical trial on humans isn't really possible to *do* on the topic. The FDA recognizes all of the sugar substitutes on the market these days as "generally recognized as safe," or GRAS, meaning that in the amount that humans could *possibly, physically consume Sweet'N Low in one day*. There is simply no scientific reason why sugar substitutes could be deemed "harmful" or substances that lead to cancer. In fact, the National Cancer Institute, American Diabetes Association, and American Heart Association all agree they do not, and those are legit institutions!

All of this being said, sugar substitutes aren't necessarily, across-the-board wonderful, nor am I suggesting that you *start* drinking diet soda if you've *only* consumed water, coffee, and tea your entire life. There are a few reasons for that.

1. **Sugar substitutes and BMI:** A multitude of studies have examined possible association between sugar substitutes and BMI, and the evidence remains inconclusive—mostly because of the same types of studies we looked at in sugar: There's a similarity in the "taste and reward" neuronal pathway, but since the "reward" isn't actually delivered in sugar form, the hypothesis is that your "treat!!" signal lights up without ever having the satisfaction of the "reward." The other limitation of evaluating that theory is a key to understanding why observational studies give us mixed messages to begin with: It's difficult to find concrete clinical significance or make recommendations based on current research when we're *observing* people who drink diet soda and making public health statements based on

said observations. While studies have found a significant association between intake of sugar-free beverages and overweight BMI (and support the biological plausibility of that finding), the predominant and overarching confounder is that individuals who have higher intake of diet beverages may *also* be on a diet *to* lose weight. Therefore, long-term weight gain and higher BMI may be a result of decreased satiety and compensatory mechanisms for energy restriction, rather than diet beverage intake.

2. **Sugar substitutes and appetite:** Remember at the beginning of this chapter when we talked about taste-and-reward mechanisms being activated when you taste something sweet? A new body of research is showing a *possible* link between drinking something sweet-tasting—triggering sweet "sensors" in your neurological system—but not getting the delight of the "reward," a loop from hell that scientists have linked to making you "crave" more sugar because your body never had the satisfaction experience of getting the actual sugar to metabolize. That said, this is a theory, not a finding—despite all the reporting on the topic! We still don't know if people eat sweets as a direct result of drinking or eating a sugar substitute, or if they drink and eat sweets and feel better about doing so *because* they had a diet beverage.

3. **Sugar substitutes and cancer:** Because of some of the hyperbolic media coverage regarding bladder cancer in rats in the 1970s, saccharin, aspartame, sucralose, and acesulfame-K are a few of the most commonly used sugar substitutes on the market that have come under some serious scrutiny for their potential role in the pathophysiology of certain types of cancers—and created a whole lot of stigma surrounding use of said substitutes. That being said, sugar substitutes have been "one of those foods" that gain traction for being "poison" for absolutely zero scientific *reason*: The study performed on rat models receiving saccharin throughout their life span was later found to be unsafe for *rats only* (in other words, according to the National Cancer Institute, "not relevant to humans"). As for aspartame, a 2005 study got everyone fired up again unnecessarily—a flawed, misreported study claimed that aspartame administered

in very high doses could cause lymphoma in rats, but this was also unfounded and a pathophysiology that applies only to *genetically modified mice*. Last, one of my favorite sugar substitutes, sucralose, gets a terrible reputation for a reason that is unknown to me (one 2016 study conducted by the same lab as the aspartame study found that it could cause blood cell tumors in mice, but the study was also shut down by FDA scientists, who found profound flaws in its evaluation methods). Splenda also has the sugar lobby against it because it can be used far more efficiently in baking than other types of sugar substitutes, while still behaving from a food chemistry standpoint the way sugar does (so you can imagine how that makes them unhappy). Why do I call sucralose my top choice in this category? You can use less of it for a more powerful effect, and it's backed by 110 scientific safety studies to make absolute *sure* it was GRAS before being officially approved for general use in 2016.

With all of this science, I completely understand why you could look at the same exact data that I'm looking at and make the choice to *not use sugar substitutes*. And hey! That's okay with me. (Remember, this is the judgment-free zone, people!) The jury is still out on the very-long-term effects of consuming super high doses of non-nutritive sweeteners over a prolonged period of time, since all of these substitutes have been approved for general use on the market and GRAS by the FDA from the 1970s on (meaning they're still *new*, considering that sugar's been around since the beginning of time). But here's the bottom line: Many people who are opposed to non-nutritive sweeteners out of concern over long-term health benefits are often concerned about this chronic disease component—a theory that's been essentially rendered baseless since the inception of these compounds. My bottom line: If you're not into sugar subs because they give you a headache, upset your tummy, or simply give you pause—that's just fine with me! But I don't want you avoiding things because you unnecessarily think they're unsafe for you, okay?

Sweetener	Regulatory Status	Examples of Brand Names Containing Sweetener	Multiplier of Sweetness Intensity Compared to Table Sugar (Sucrose)	Acceptable Daily Intake (ADI), milligrams per kilogram body weight per day (mg/kg bw/d)	Number of Tabletop Sweetener Packets Equivalent to ADI
Acesulfame potassium (Acesulfame-K)	Approved as a sweetener and flavor enhancer in foods generally (except in meat and poultry)	Sweet One Sunett	200x	15	23
Advantame	Approved as a sweetener and flavor enhancer in foods generally (except in meat and poultry)		20,000x	32.8	4,920
Aspartame	Approved as a sweetener and flavor enhancer in foods generally	NutraSweet Equal Sugar Twin	200x	50	75
Neotame	Approved as a sweetener and flavor enhancer in foods generally (except meat and poultry)	Newtame	7,000–13,000x	0.3	23 (sweetness intensity at 10,000x sucrose)
Saccharin	Approved as a sweetener only in certain special dietary foods and as an additive used for certain technological purposes	Sweet'N Low Sweet Twin Sweet and Low Necta Sweet	200–700x	15	45 (sweetness intensity at 400x sucrose)
Siraitia grosvenorii Swingle (Luo Han Guo) fruit extracts (SGFE)	SGFE containing 25%, 45%, or 55% mogroside V is the subject of GRAS notices for specific conditions of use	Truvia PureVita Enliten	200–400x	4	9 (sweetness intensity at 300x sucrose)
Sucralose	Approved as a sweetener in foods generally	Splenda	600x	5	23

TESTING THE SAFETY OF NON-NUTRITIVE SWEETENERS

The amount of non-nutritive sweeteners given to animals in order to test for safety is purposefully dosed at amounts *significantly higher* per kilogram of body weight than humans will likely be exposed to—simply for this reason: to make sure that ingesting them in any amount even remotely conceivable to humans is safe. For example, the acceptable daily intake (ADI) of aspartame in the United States is 50 milligrams per kilogram of body weight; in the EU, it is slightly lower (40 mg per kilogram). How does that translate (as per the American Cancer Society)? To put the U.S. ADI for aspartame in perspective, this would be 3,750 mg per day for a typical adult weighing 75 kilograms (about 165 pounds)—far more than most adults take in daily. A can of diet soda usually contains about 180 mg of aspartame, so a typical adult would have to drink about 21 cans of diet soda a day to go over the recommended level—and even *that* would have to be done consistently over the course of time in order to reach the amount that puts you at risk for chronic disease.

(*Shout-out to Sally in Sacramento drinking 22 cans of sugar-free soda: You're just one over the limit, girl. DO LESS.*)

Does Eating Sugar Raise My Chance of Diabetes?

Unless you become clinically obese, eating a lot of sugar does not *directly* put you at risk for diabetes. That said, diets high in saturated fats and added sugars are linked to an increased risk of developing type 2 diabetes, as well as heart disease and some lifestyle-related cancers. That's because if you're eating anything in excess of what your body needs, your organs will, over time, desensitize or change in DNA composition (something that your genes also play a role in determining—your level of susceptibility to overconsumption of these nutrients). It is also worth noting that the higher your diet is in sugar, the lower your diet is in things that can help *protect you* against chronic disease. Think about it this way—if you're surviving on sugar (baked goods, sugary bevs, sugary cereals, and chocolate—*only*), then what are you likely *not eating in the course of a day*? Antioxidants, in the form of vegetables, fruit, whole grains, beans/legumes, nuts, and seeds—and even your protein sources, too, provide a whole bunch of great-for-you nutrients (especially seafood). So there you are, eating lots of fried food dipped in sugar, and your liver is becoming a little tired of this deep-fried-brownie-at-every-meal scenario. Your pancreas is firing off insulin at every turn, and your cells *are* overflowing in sugar, taking it up and storing it in your peripheral tissues, time after time after time. Eventually, everything's going to get a little worn out—especially when your cells have no defenses to use for protection against advanced glycation end products (AGEs), which are basically the sugar-metabolism edition of cholesterol deposits in your blood vessels (i.e., plaque). And guess what? You have no defenses readily available, because you're not eating all of the antioxidants from the best foods in the world! It's these scenarios that show you just how powerful it is to eat more of the good stuff, rather than talking so much about "elimination" or "cutting back." If you have no defenses, your organs can't really fight back in a way that helps keep *you free of chronic disease*!

Bottom line: You might see an Instagram picture of donuts captioned "OMG these are so worth the diabetes!" But that's just plain wrong, wrong, wrong. You can troll them, if you like—you have my permission.

What's the Glycemic Index? (And Do I Need to Know About It?)

The glycemic index refers to a measure of how a particular amount of carbohydrate affects blood sugar. It can change based on which foods you combine together. For example, a plain baked potato is considered a higher GI food, but when you add sour cream, cheese, bacon, and beans, it's a super low GI food (and a little rough on the GI tract, I might add...). For our purposes, though, I think it's a misused term, because it makes people think it has something to do with nutritional quality of a food when you say "low glycemic index," and it's often used as a marketing term on food labels these days (and what *isn't*, am I right?!). But as you can see by our baked potato example, loads of cheddar and cream do not a "super-nutritious food" product make. Conversely, most nutritionally excellent foods *are* low GI, like beans, for example. That's because they've got fiber and plant protein (the part that takes time to digest and absorb), but they're also antioxidant- and mineral-packed (the part that contributes to their general greatness).

High-GI foods: pretzels, candy, potatoes, sweet potatoes, and white bread, like bagels.

Low-GI foods: 100% whole grains, al dente pasta and rice, berries, leafy greens, like kale.

(Source: The American Diabetes Association website, accessed June 2018.)

Bottom line: It's a great term if you're an athlete, because you need some high-GI foods before you go for a long training run. For the rest of us: This is one you can (mostly) ignore.

Brown Sugar Versus Refined Sugar

No one cares, Doris. One isn't less processed than the other. Marketers use *refined* as a buzzword, because language surrounding "refined carbo-hydrates" is ubiquitous, so if anyone is able to promote the "wholesome quality" of their sugar-containing product, they're going to jump on any opportunity to do so. Brown sugar versus white sugar versus refined sugar, though, is all from the same place—sugarcane. And it'll all be metabolized just the same.

Is Honey Considered Sugar? What About Agave?

Yes, which is *confusing* if you're a chemist thinking in terms of the nuanced chemical structures of each. But *not* if you're a consumer (which most of you *are. Yay!*). According to the FDA:

The sugar in a jar of honey and the sugar in a bag of sugar are added sugars. The definition of added sugars includes sugars that are either added during the processing of foods, or are packaged as such, and include sugars (free, mono- and disaccharides), sugars from syrups and honey.

Honey, just like agave nectar and maple syrup, and lots of other sneaky syrups (tapioca, brown rice, corn, sorghum, dextrose, wheat, and glucose, to name just a few...) are all still concentrated forms of sugar.

Is Stevia an Artificial Sweetener?

It's not "artificial" by the FDA's definition, but I wouldn't call it the picture of wholesome, either—I mean, it's not kale. Since stevia is made from a plant extract (*Stevia rebaudiana* or stevioside) that's been refined, it falls under the FDA designation of "natural"—the effects of which have manifested across food products that use stevia as a sweetener and also use the term "no artificial sweetener" (while the other artificial sweeteners are made from compounds that are distant cousins of plants or are entirely man-made). This is another nebulous one, because the crude stevia leaf itself is not considered GRAS, and the FDA *doesn't* import the actual raw plant for use as a sweetener. The take-home here: Stevia has 0 grams of sugar, just as the artificial types do. Some people like stevia as an alternative to sweeteners because it's thought of as better tolerated for the tummy, but critics consider the taste to have a profound lingering effect on your tongue (ick).

Ultimately, the choice is yours on which ones to use and when to use 'em.

Aren't Some Low-, Reduced-, or Fat-Free Products Really Full of Sugar?!

Yep. (Bummer—this is tough, isn't it?! It'll be easy in a sec.) Case in point, words matter on the sugar topic. But in foods that contain multiple ingredients as a part of recipe development and ingredient-processing—that's a horse of an entirely *different color*. Let's break it down.

Dry snacks (chips, crackers, pretzels, popcorn, and various iterations of all of those) use oil in order to fry or bake the tasty, crunchy lil' snack and follow an ingredient "formula" (dare I call this a *recipe*?!) in order to be made consistently (this now includes doing fancy things like using machines). In the 1980s and '90s, when food marketers really took advantage of the whole "cut back on dietary fat and cholesterol" thing, the food industry took this concept seriously and ran with it. Low-fat refrigerated desserts (anyone else have packaged pudding as a mainstay in their family home growing up?) and frozen desserts; low-fat cookies, low-fat cream, whipped cream, and flavored milks—pretty much everything you could ever want to eat was suddenly available with a low-fat claim slapped on the front of the pack.

What happens when you remove the fat from something that's already made with added sugar? You need something to replace the tasty, creamy, filling flavor of fat. So those savvy manufacturers turned up the sugar in order to pull back on the fat content. The end result: A product that's about the same (maybe a few less) in total calories, but lower in fat and higher in sugar.

Bottom line: Your guideline for lower fat with higher sugar, and vice versa, should be related to how much of the food you plan on using. For example: A sweetened Greek yogurt like the Fage we keep coming back to is a *better* choice than a venti vanilla latte because in the latter, you're going to add upward of 40 grams of sugar based on size alone.

#protip

The same goes for nonfat, fat-free, full-fat, and part-skim products: If you're going to use a lot of it, nonfat might be a better choice for you. But if you're using a little bit (like me and my half-and-half—you can't separate me from that stuff in my coffee!), opt for the real deal. When it comes to cheeses: Mixing nonfat and whole together is often what I recommend in practice, because people typically have both types on hand for different purposes. They make for a nice, limited-in-saturated-fat (but not totally tasteless!) topping, no matter what you're making.

Added Sugar by the Aisle

Crackers and chips

Sneaky, but these are often sweetened. Check labels for savory products under 2 grams of sugar (if they're plain flavored), and under 4 grams if they're a flavor that's designed to make them taste a specific way (e.g., barbecue sauce).

Snack bars

First things first: If you're aiming to cut back on added sugar but *also* make a more nutritious, wholesome choice that closely resembles *real food*, you want that first ingredient to be a real food—nuts are usually the most nutritious first ingredient in a good-for-you bar, but a fruit or a 100 percent whole grain will also do the trick.

Next, look for a satisfying combo of protein and fiber, plus some fat, and an added sugar value that's under 6–8 grams (depending on your use—remember 8 grams is "acceptable" if you're using this product as your dessert, but less great if you want to eat it to tide you over between meals). For snack products, the lowest I ever recommend going on each is 4 grams fiber and 4 grams protein (you know this already from chapter 6!). But I specify those nutrients in our conversation about sugar because—little-known fact—as someone who spends most days evaluating consumer food products and analyzing ingredients/labels, I can speak confidently about the fact that for the *most part*, you're automatically cutting out a class of highly sugary foods by making 3 grams your baseline. Make 4 grams an even *better* goal to help guide you to more nutritious choices. Bottom line: Regardless of the Nutrition Facts label (old versus new), it's a good rule of thumb to make sugar under 10 g your goal. Otherwise, go for 4 g each protein and fiber for more filling snacks to keep up energy and boost satiety between meals. Choose bars with a minimum of 3 g each protein and fiber for a nutritious option when there's not much else that's available to you, or you're purposefully looking for something smaller to tide you over till your *next* meal.

Fruit-based condiments and syrups

As a general guideline, these will all rank around 15 grams for a 2-tablespoon serving of sugary syrup, which is why they rack up so quickly. Looking for lower-sugar options is a great way to cut sugar if these are household staples, but you can also do this yourself by using less and considering other ways to add extra flavor. Case in point: A serving of jelly has 15 grams sugar, but this is one where you're not likely to be using the full serving (2 tablespoons). One teaspoon (4 g, or 1 teaspoon of sugar) goes a long way for you in flavor—especially if you bought, say, raspberry preserves, add a teaspoon of jelly to your PB&J, and smush in about ½ cup of raspberries to complete that meal with extra fiber. If you're flavoring up griddle cakes like pancakes, French toast, or waffles (the real kind, folks), think about adding in some sweetness from a veggie or fruit source, like pumpkin puree in waffles, pancakes, and toast. Adding cinnamon sugar as a flavoring instead of straight sugar will also help cut back in this department, since the bottle itself is halved with cinnamon.

Condiments and dressings

Choose naturally flavor-boosting toppings instead, like salsas, hot sauce, or mashed avocado (aka guac!) and swap Greek yogurt or cottage cheese for higher-fat dips made from cream, and you'll be good to go without all of the sneaky sweet stuff. That said, if you are a dressing aficionado, look for ones that provide 4 grams or less of added sugar per serving, and under 250 milligrams sodium. Truth: If you couldn't tell already by the name of this book, grocery shopping to seek out a bottle of salad dressing is somewhat elusive to me.

Nut butters and spreads

Aim for sugar to hover around 6 grams or less in a *flavored nut butter* (plain versions should have 0 grams), like versions with fruit or chocolate mixed in. But more important is that the ingredients list is pretty simple on this one. Much more than that, and it's a real dessert, in which case make sure you're choosing one of these items for the intention of eating it as a treat—not as fuel to power through (which PB is otherwise!).

Sauce

BBQ sauce, ketchup, and tomato sauce can be sneaky culprits of added sugar—½ cup of BBQ sauce has up to 10 grams of added sugar, and sweetened tomato sauce can go up to 15. Ketchup, too, is 4 grams per tablespoon. Look for lower-sugar or reduced-sugar alternatives for all of these, but swapping BBQ sauce for dry rub (or using less *with* a dry rub), using tomato paste (unsweetened) in place of ketchup, and looking for sauces without sugar in the ingredients list will lend a hand.

Dairy products

- Aim to keep yogurt at no more than 12 grams of *total sugar* per serving when it's a part of a meal or you're eating it as a snack on its own. (Heads-up, readers: This is going to be a little tough for you at time of publication, because there aren't that many on the market that are flavored, tasty, *and* 12 grams or less!) Look for Chobani Pumpkin Spice or Siggi's Dairy, and consider buying plain versions that you can sweeten on your own or flavor with spices. Pumpkin pie spice = pumpkin puree + cinnamon + nutmeg + a drizzle of a non-nutritive sweetener or honey: It is super delicious and will make you wonder why you ever considered flavored yogurt a satisfying choice to begin with! Cottage cheese is similar, and most are under 10 grams regardless.

- Flavored milk (like chocolate milk) should cap total sugar at 16 grams—that's a teaspoon above what's already in there naturally.
- Plant-based milks should have 0 grams of added sugar as often as possible. Remember, cow's milk has 12 grams of naturally occurring sugar, but it's also got 8 grams of protein. The other types of plant milks consider sugar "added," since there won't be any in there naturally (almonds don't have sugar on their own, people!). So unless vanilla almond milk is *truly* your sugar of choice for the day, look for plain versions to cut back where you can.

CEREAL SMARTS

Without question, the food that's gotten the most flack in the media for its opaque nutritional attributes is sweetened cereal. (Real talk: If Tony the Tiger were trying to survive in his natural habitat on flakes of frosted corn flour, there's no chance he would've been strong enough to stand up to other predators, am I right?). I think cereal is just glorious, if we consider it for *what it actually is: Breakfast*, when it's plain, unsweetened, and made from 100 percent whole grains. It's *dessert* when it's frosted, fruity, chocolate, glazed, crunchy, or claims to be modeled after a more indulgent breakfast item—for example, pancakes, French toast, or waffles (c'mon—you *all know* what I'm talking about!). Think of it this way: Any food can have a *place* in your diet, if you love sweet cereal and want to use something sweet and delicious as a topping or as a treat, well, *grrreeat*! The confusing part is where these cereals "live" in the grocery store (often *next to* the foods that are otherwise more nutrient-dense, and far from the bakery). Some tips:

- Check that ingredients list before you buy and look for real food. Start with things that are 100 percent whole grain or a real food as the first ingredient (whole-grain oats, wheat, almonds...you see where we're going with this!) and then look for as few ingredients as possible—then you can spice it up with your own real food like fruits, and more.

    Look for a minimum of 3 grams each protein and fiber, with major bonus points if the product has a significant amount (more than 6 g of protein, more than 9 g of fiber). Keep in mind that ½ cup of Greek yogurt has about 10 grams of protein, while ½ cup of regular or skim milk has 4 grams protein (plant-based alternatives like almond or coconut milk are 0 g).

    Often, cereal marketing plays up their best attributes (e.g., "good source of fiber, good source of vitamin C"), but since you can get your fill of good-for-you nutrients from better sources throughout the day, it's more important to look at added sugar, saturated fat, sodium, and the ingredients list on the whole rather than singling out one nutrient.

Okay, If I Cut Back on the Sugar...What Can I Have Now?!

There are times when you just want to eat some sweets, and you don't care where they come from. Consider that when it comes to treats you bring *into* your home *from the grocery store*—more special treats that come from certain bakeries, dessert bars, or restaurants that we'll cover later on. For now, let's talk about the greatest food on the planet, *candy*. It's sugar in its happiest form, and isn't (usually) trying to be something it's not. (*Respect!*) Here are some guidelines involved in "going for it":

- **Max out at 250 calories per serving.** Look for options that are 150–250 calories or less per serving. Options with nuts (peanuts, almonds) are higher in fat, but as a result, they're often more satisfying—they'll provide a little bit of protein and fiber (peanut M&M's, for example, are 5 g protein and 2 g fiber at 240 calories per pack).

■ **When in doubt, choose chocolate.** Chocolate candies are (typically) a better nutritional choice because they, too, are more satisfying than sour/gummy candies, which are straight sugar. Chocolate itself is higher in fat and feels a little bit more indulgent, so it can make it just a little bit harder to "overdo." Your general nutrition goals: Some items are better than others, so let 20 g sugar be your max, and on the whole, aim to keep saturated fat and sodium as low as possible when choosing between items.

■ **Reminder: Don't be swayed by lame claims.** If you actually find a whole, fresh strawberry walking out of your pack of Starburst... something's wrong. They're not harmful to eat in their prepackaged amounts, but just be wary of claims on processed foods—it doesn't indicate that something is "more nutritious." Another one to watch: "low-fat." Gummy candies will also make this claim, which is true (many contain 0 g fat), but since they're often consumed as excess calories (you're not *really* having Swedish fish for lunch, right?), they'll *still* be "stored" if the energy they provide is in surplus of what you *need*.

#protip

Pick two to three bags of your favorite individually wrapped candies (different types or flavors per bag—not mixed bags), which is enough to make your whole family (or just you!) happy.

- **Empty the bags and store in the freezer in a container.** This helps you take them out in serving size, let them thaw, and enjoy when you're going for a treat. It also builds in a pause before you go back for more: You'll have that whole "unwrapping," "thawing" time to decide if you really want it—or if it's not worth the wait.

- **Consider quality over quantity:** You know this one, but there's some additional nuance to it in this context. For example: There's a difference in taste between brands of certain types of candies. In practice, hard candies and lollipops go a long way for many of my clients, when you *just need something sweet*. They're sweet, long-lasting, and often available in flavors that totally *satisfy*, which is why I recommend looking for specific flavors, brands, or store-specific items (personally, that's a See's Candies cinnamon lollipop; *but, Steve, I know how you love getting to the center of that grape Tootsie Pop—have at it!*). Items that take longer to consume *also* play point guard for you in a subtler way: The time you take to enjoy a little sweetness provides you with a built-in pause to digest and absorb, meaning you're more likely to register satiety instead of diving back into the mac and cheese. Some other great ones:

Prepackaged minis: Prepackaged ice cream pops, like a mini Klondike or a mini Häagen-Dazs cup, are all better options than bringing the whole icy tub into your home and feeling like the ice cream is calling to you from the freezer. (Mini Magnum, which is the size of the real deal of most other types of ice cream; Good Humor Strawberry Shortcake bars; Blue Bunny Mini Cones; and Trader Joe's Hold the Cone are great picks for this, too.)

Bulk candies that are *just chocolate*: Dove and Hershey's do this best: You can have *nine* Hershey's Kisses to yield a full serving! For volume-lovers, this is a great moment to go for it consciously rather than mindlessly.

Cinnamon of any kind: If it's spicy enough, you'll slow down as you go. See's lollipops, cinnamon fireballs, and hot tamales have all been a successful treat option with clients. The tamales (and their less spicy version in the form of Mike and Ike's) are extra delicious and slower to eat when you opt for 'em straight out of the freezer, too.

Single-serve chocolate-covered fruit: Diana's Bananas and Dole Dippers make "dipped in chocolate" fruit items that come in their own packages. There's lots of items like these on the market (you'll find many at Trader Joe's, too).

Mint, peppermint, and all of its derivatives: Peppermint patties and Andes mints are another idea for getting you to naturally cut back on sugar. That's because you're primed to eat *less* overall when you go for the real thing, but won't want to spoil that fresh flavor by going for something *else*.

Dark chocolate—and not for the "antioxidants": Along the lines of "making it fancy" to make it last: Getting a specialty type of super-rich dark chocolate or chocolates from somewhere *amazing*—a local chocolate shop, a candy store you love that's tough to get to—is a bit self-limiting.

Candy's Okay, but I Really Love Ice Cream. Am I Out of Luck?

Ice cream is fun! But you know what's more fun? Gelato. It's great because it's the same indulgent treat as ice cream, but often slightly lower in calories and sugar thanks to the fact that it's made with more milk and less cream. Per serving, you'll wind up cutting the calories by about 30 percent without feeling like you went without. This is my recommendation over something like frozen yogurt, which is loaded with added sugar and, calorie-wise, often the exact same as, if not more than, regular ice cream—but it won't feel like it, because it's missing the filling fat.

The question I'm getting more than ever, though, is about the "new" face of diet ice cream. Yes—you can eat the whole pint in a given night if that's your real, tried and true dessert of about 250 calories (that's your standard Halo Top version). But for many of us, this (a) won't be our only sweet treat in a day, and (b) isn't necessarily your most satisfying option because it's made from nonfat milk as the first ingredient (or a plant-based, processed-out-the-fat milk like coconut) and contains lots of sugar alcohols. "Healthy ice cream," sounds a bit like saying, "Santa Clause is real," right? The new ice creams that claim to be lower in sugar but higher in protein are made from *similar* ingredients: milk, eggs, cream, and (some) sugar. Unlike regular frozen treats, however, these newbies also contain added protein isolate, synthetic fibers, emulsifying agents, stevia, and sugar alcohols—all of which are designed to make them taste *more like ice cream*. So don't get me wrong—there's nothing wrong with eating them, but it's prudent for you to know going in that they're not as satisfying as ice cream (so don't feel like you've been robbed! They told you that on the ingredients list/Nutrition Facts label!)

and that sugar alcohols can give you gas, stomach pains from gas, bloating, and, for some, diarrhea. So, while they're lower in added sugar and saturated fat, you can enjoy them without necessarily adding a significant amount of energy onto what you need in a day. But you may also be committing to an evening on the toilet—so consider yourself warned.

The last point I want to call out here is this: They promote eating a whole container of ice cream, which is a habit I have reservations about. That can trigger a binge in those of us who are a little bit more susceptible to overeating—this may not be a *safe food* for you if you feel like it's a gate-opener! One full pint a day also isn't exactly the most cost-efficient dessert you can find.

When you swap in fake ingredients for the real ones, there's always the risk that you'll feel less satisfied—and wind up eating more overall than if you'd just gone with a smaller portion of the original stuff in the first place. My advice: Choose whichever version makes you feel more satisfied. Just keep in mind that it's still a dessert, not sustenance!

8

Postwork Drinks and Dinners Out Are a Huge Part of My Everyday Life

After this chapter, you will...

- plan pregame and postgame strategies for all drinking and dining festivities in your daily life;
- develop your own personal Ulysses contract for all dining experiences;
- devise a fallback, go-to strategy for food-related situations you're unable to avoid; and
- strategize in advance for busy workdays and unavoidable professional socializing.

Why Does Every Business Dinner Seem to Start with Bread and End with Brownies?

Going out is such a trigger point for so many people. Socializing, be it for business purposes or otherwise, tends to have the greatest level of variability. Let's compare it to something like going to the movies. When you go, the chances are pretty great that there are some highly expected options available to you: Popcorn! Soda! Candy! Chocolate! Pretzel bites with extremely yellow hot cheese! If you go out for drinks or dinner with people whom you either don't know very well, or *do know* but they're highly unpredictable, it's difficult to make a plan. Since there're loads of potential pitfalls, any given social or professional situation has the greatest perception of being "high-risk" for anxiety thanks to the greatest amount of variability.

Fears that come my way sound like this: *"There are so many places I can mess up! And this is the part of my life that probably needs the MOST help to get me to lose weight! And even if I do SO GREAT during the week, I can't change how or who I am in my free time!"* These are TDTs, of course; they're *simply untrue.*

The one thing I see consistently among clients when it comes to making behavior change around their state of health is a perception that in order to make healthier choices, you can't actually have any alcohol or do anything that even resembles having *fun.* There are two big reasons for this type of fear.

The first is the resistance to changing something that is *designed* to be fun, light, and enjoyable. *So* many clients think, *"I don't want to 'diet' while I'm having fun! I want to eat and drink and be f-ing merry! WHY WON'T YOU JUST LET ME LIVE?!"*

But, *hello?!* See why that's *toxic*? Excuse the use of this trope, but living your best life includes having fun and being able to cut loose. You want to be able to make healthier choices a reasonable, manageable, and sustainable part of your everyday lifestyle, not to eliminate them completely or make you feel like you have up until right now. I'm either being "good" or I'm "boozing it up" with colleagues is a false paradigm—those things can't live in their own perfect silos, but they also aren't mutually exclusive. In order to live your life and do your job, you have to be able to manage both in a way that feels health-focused and health-promoting for *you.* It's true that this will mean you have to make sacrifices in some areas so that you can achieve bigger goals in other areas. But you have every right to change your mind at any time about how to handle yourself—you just have to set up your own Ulysses contract for managing these moments so that you can do all of *that* without feeling like you're not being kind enough to numero uno (aka *you*; chapter 4, anyone?!).

Lessons from an Astronaut

My client, whom we'll call Alice, is a highly successful lawyer in New York City. She is an awesome single woman who dates, goes out with friends, entertains coworkers, and manages an aggressive schedule, both in and out of court. Alice also goes to a number of different exercise classes a week, and she's never afraid to try something new. She's confident, strong, hilariously funny, and takes absolutely zero bullsh*t from her clients (or her opponents, of course). To my knowledge, there is only one person in Alice's life that she's ever taken bs from—and that is *herself*. Alice came in to see me at the recommendation of her endocrinologist, who had suggested a change in Alice's eating habits in order to lose weight and perhaps offset Alice's need to start taking blood-sugar-controlling medication. Prediabetes and type 2 diabetes run in her family—her grandparents, both parents, and older sister were all on medication for management of it, so to her, it felt almost inevitable to start taking meds for better blood sugar control. In her early forties, Alice had been the walking definition of "YOLO": She wanted to lose weight, but she also felt like skipping out on eating and drinking whatever she wanted all of the time was antithetical to having a fulfilled life.

Alice had a mental block around weight loss and changing her habits. I was pretty sure it was because she knew there was a fallback plan in place: If she didn't lose weight in a few months, she'd go on metformin, an oral hypoglycemic that's taken by many with type 2 diabetes. So *why* would Alice come and seek counseling from yours truly if she could be taking a drug that could just do all of this stuff—blood sugar control and weight loss—*for* her? Clearly, she wanted to explore what else was out there—at age 41, she wasn't particularly psyched to start taking a medication that she might need to be on for the rest of her life.

When Alice came in, she and I would talk about her week, and I would give her a plan specific to her set of circumstances. It would sound something like this: "You're going to see the new John Cena movie? Here's what you'll eat while you're at the theater. Are you going to that tapas bar in NoMad this week? This is what to order. Are you having family dinner at that seafood restaurant on Friday? Have the calamari grilled instead of fried, start with the chopped salad, and split the salmon with your niece—YOU CAN GET THE *FRIED* CALAMARI NEXT TIME, I PROMISE!"

Alice would come back the next week and show me a food journal with literally every food item I'd asked her *not* to order. (Sounds like a dream client, huh?)

Finally, I just called her out on it.

"If I gave you a mapped-out meal plan for what to eat on the moon, you would come back to me next week and tell me you last-minute decided to go to Mars instead. You're basically an astronaut. It's like, I'm NASA over here telling you what to do when you get to space, and you're like, *What do you know, Houston?! I'll do what I want!*"

She and I had a good laugh about it, but calling her attention to the scenario-driven, "what to eat, *when*" context of my plans for her actually wound up resonating. The scenario-driven, "eat-this-when-you-get-here" concept was still the key to helping her make changes, but we hadn't been tackling a key part of the scenario: the associations Alice had between an activity, the food, and above all else, *the drinks*.

Alice associated a variety of restaurants, eating occasions, festive events, and celebrations with one type of beverage and one type of meal. When she ordered X beverage, she would eat Y with it—*period*. In her self-designed eating plan, she would order, say, a margarita—and then always order the nachos along with it—simply because changing *that* part of her habit and adjusting that pattern, in that order, felt too disappointing and completely unsatisfying all at once. I'd previously been thinking that limiting Alice to just one of her favorite beverages was the best place to start for her—one thing at a time, better food choices shouldn't be an automatic buzzkill, and all that. But she didn't want to just have *one* frozen margarita! She wanted two, and she wanted to be able to have the nachos with it, *dammit, Jackie*!!

So the problem was that Alice was stuck in her fixed patterns of beverage and food associations. Once we identified the fact that it all began with the margarita itself (that frozen cocktails = nachos to Alice), I was able to come up with a new way forward.

I asked her to start with the booze: She could still have two margs—maybe even three if she wanted, but they couldn't be frozen and pre-mixed. Instead, she would order some great, pricey Patrón or silver tequila with *tons* of fresh-squeezed lime juice and a splash of triple sec on the rocks. She tried it, and the results were terrific. When she ordered one she liked and left the option open to have another (and maybe *another*), two things happened: First, she sipped slower, because the drink was stronger. This one change—swapping one thing she liked for another thing she liked that was just a little different—got her down about 2 pounds our first week. She really liked that and was inspired to change something else about the order. "Instead of nachos, I did what you actually said to do," she said casually at our next week's meeting. "I ordered the steak fajitas with extra veggies, plus guac and salsa—it was delicious! I want to have that every night now."

Well, what do you know! Alice was down 5 pounds the following week. Once she started to use these tools—tangibly making adjustments to the beverage and keeping the flavors but switching up the preparation of her favorite food pairings, she wound up losing a total of 40 pounds in the six months we worked together. At one of our last sessions, I asked her what part of working together had helped light a fire under her. Her response was ideal: "Nothing, really," she said. "At first it seemed like you were trying to take food away from me, but I realized I actually eat way more than I used to and I drink about the same—maybe a little bit less, but I drink the good stuff now! I just didn't completely see that the cocktails were my own gate-keeper for making better food choices."

Now, Alice is, in her words, "at my high-school weight!" and living her life in all kinds of expansive, risk-taking ways that don't ever make her feel trapped or like she's "dieting."

This type of transition from complete overwhelm and resistance isn't unique to Alice (although she *is* pretty special as far as human beings go—*love you, girl!*). It's so common, in fact, that it's got a psychology name (*of course it does*): it's called "stages of change." It refers to addiction behavior change but is easily applied in a model of weight loss and health management, too. When a person is in the early stages of change, called precontemplation, they need to do a little experimentation to see what kinds of changes feel appealing, sustainable, and manageable. Alice went from a precontemplative "I'm overwhelmed, but I'm thinking about making a change and I'm seeing a dietitian instead of going straight to the meds" to "I tried one thing, and now I'm doing all kinds of great things that help me eat better—and it's working!"

The Transtheoretical Model of Behavior Change

Behavior Change Stages and Their Characteristics	
Stage	**Characteristics**
Precontemplation	Individual does not intend to change behavior in the next six months.
Contemplation	Individual is strongly inclined to change behavior in the next six months.
Preparation	Individual intends to act in the near future (generally next month).
Action	Behavior has already been incorporated for at least six months.
Maintenance	Action already happens for over six months and the chances to return to old behavior are few.

This model is a big one for RDs, because there is often the assumption among clients that by simply showing up to a consultation, they will magically lose weight. I wish it were that simple! Unlike physicians, who can prescribe a medication and see immediate results, nutritionists are banking on the fact that those who seek our help will apply our feedback, and it's up to us to employ motivational interviewing to encourage clients to identify what is holding them back from making changes that work for them. The way that clients come to this realization, however, takes many different paths. Once we identify barriers to change, it's easier to start making progress. Knowing your own beliefs and how they stop you from or propel you toward making changes is the single greatest challenge.

Determine Your Goals and Objectives

The first plan of action when you know a happy hour is upon you: Know your goals and objectives (yes, I'm serious…). If you know what you're looking to get *out of the hour* (or few hours, in many cases), you'll know how to strategize what to eat and drink in more specific terms. Here, we'll go through each goal: Socializing, meeting with a superior or boss, and what to do when you're just trying to get in and out in under thirty minutes. We'll then go through what's available in most of these post-office hour scenarios; what to drink and eat specifically (how to make it dinner versus how to make it a pre-dinner snack); what you should snack on when there's no food available; what to choose (and why) for at-the-bar nosh; and how to set yourself up for success when you're sharing apps, meals, and pitchers with coworkers.

Honestly, the worst part about eating healthfully has nothing to do with making nutritious meals at home. (If I only ever ate at home, I'd have no problem with maintaining a healthful diet!) No, the absolute worst part is feeling like you have no clue what to order when you're out with your friends or on a date—something that likely happens at least a time or two a week for all of us. *One restaurant meal* has us eating most of the calories, fat, and sodium we need in one day. But what if you had an RD to help highlight the tricky ordering pitfalls hidden on restaurant menus?

Pregame with Snacks

One hour to thirty minutes before you go to "happy hour" or any event at which you know you'll be drinking, you need a substantial snack or a true-to-form sneal. I don't care if you had a crumbly "For Sharing" cracker from Diane's desk an hour ago, or if you're on your way out of a meeting and making a beeline for the bar. You always need to have a snack on your physical person (ladies, that's in your bag; gents, that bag of almonds doubles nicely as a pocket-square!) in order to make sure you're prepped to go into any drinking scenario.

If you're aiming to make the better choice for your health or your weight, the only way you're really going to make better choices once you're confronted with the glorious chocolate fountain is to actually have prepared *enough* in advance that you're feeling *satisfied* to *not* be tempted to dive in. And because of your pregame, you're also primed to simply feel *less hungry*, so that if you did want to have a taste, you'd literally have just that—a bite or two, and feel just dandy about it. No deprivation or willpower required— you're *satisfied*! You had a snack at the pregame!

Recap: Pregame with a snack that combines protein and fiber and errs on the side of indulgent, to ward off the times when you think you might be tempted by indulgences *later on in the night*.

Go Hard on the Veg Order

The easiest, most self-limiting guideline is to remember that no matter where you are, you want most of your "plate" (at least 50 percent) to be vegetable-based. Whether that means adding extra greens on the side, starting with salad and making sure your main *also* includes veggies (and sorry, in this case potatoes don't count…) or adding extra veggies to a pasta dish, racking up the fiber content will help you feel fuller, faster—AND stay that way! It will also help you feel satisfied for the REST of your meal so that you can make better choices overall—and actually notice when you start to feel full.

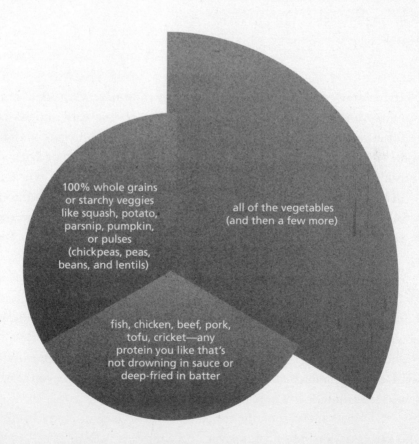

100% whole grains or starchy veggies like squash, potato, parsnip, pumpkin, or pulses (chickpeas, peas, beans, and lentils)

all of the vegetables (and then a few more)

fish, chicken, beef, pork, tofu, cricket—any protein you like that's not drowning in sauce or deep-fried in batter

Food Prep Protocol

The number one pitfall my clients run into is choosing options that would *otherwise* be healthful, but instead have high calories from fat because of the way the food is prepared. Some culprits include tempura, chicken tenders, coconut shrimp, and dumplings that aren't labeled as steamed. I always tell clients to be on the lookout for words like *crispy, crunchy, deep-fried, pan-fried, stir-fried, breaded, Parmesan, doughy/dumpling, rolls* (e.g., spring rolls, unless they're in rice paper!), or *creamy*—which all mean added calories from oil, breading, or both! Instead, your best options are steamed, grilled, roasted, broiled, boiled, poached, "lightly" sautéed, or pan seared or blackened, which can, for the most part, ensure that you're eliminating some of the added butter/oil/sauce/cream/breading and sticking to just the bare bones of the meat.

#protip

If you're not the biggest lover of veggies right now: Consider using more tomato-based sauces, ordering this at restaurants, and asking for a tomato-based soup as a starter—it's a nice little gateway veg for getting used to different ways to eat delicious produce without relying on a sad salad with "dressing on the side." (Veggie, chicken, or beef-based broths can help you get there too—e.g., hot and sour soup; tomato and basil soup; miso with veggie soup; pho with extra veggies; ramen with extra veggies, and so on.)

All About Your Drink Order

Calories from alcohol consumed while eating out can easily blunder an otherwise healthful meal—especially if you're having more than one. Rather than reaching for mixed drinks, fruit-based cocktails, or anything with tonic (e.g., margaritas, gin and tonic, mojitos, etc.)—choose the clears: wine (red, white, or champagne), spirit + soda (seltzer or diet cola—no tonic!), or the hard stuff on the rocks. This will keep calories to a minimum and also limit the double-hangover of feeling the residual effects of these high-sugar beverages (about 100–150 calories per serving). You could also try a spirit + splash of a more concentrated flavor via syrup: grenadine, cassis, elderflower, Cointreau, or lavender.

On the other hand, skip frozen drinks; margaritas; drinks with literally any sugary mixer (tonic water, regular soda, regular energy drinks, margarita mix, fruit-flavored drink mixers, drinks with juice—yes, even 100 percent all-natural juice); and even drinks with clear sodas that *seem* like they're innocuous: Ginger ale, regular Sprite, and fancy-sounding names like "ginger beer" are still going to be calorie-containing.

#protip

Ask about flavors that sound like "ingredients."

Ginger, blueberry, banana, coconut, cinnamon—these fruits and spices are often found in their syrup form when you're at a restaurant, so ask if it's fresh or if it's a syrup to clarify. You can always ask for "less" or "a drop of" instead of going all in, or see if you can order that drink with a fresh alternative—herbs, fresh ginger, and jalapeno are *dee-licious*!

If you *are opting* for the occasional sugary bev, then okay—your plan is to have one, and switch to something else immediately after. If you're committing to weight loss, eating calories versus drinking them is one of the more important choices you can make *right now*. (And why not give this a trial run STAT?) We'll talk about this more in the next chapter, but if we're going to start, why not start now? Plus, the other benefit of cutting back on calories from beverages: The trade-off is the equivalent of dessert, which you can now *actually eat*. (*You're welcome*.)

Have a Restaurant-Specific Ulysses Contract

Here you are, at your local steak house, and you were all geared up to order yourself some "petit filet," side of veggies, and the grilled artichoke. But, bad news—they're out of petit filet! And the starter salad special today is

CHEESY TATER TOTS WITH EXTRA BACON AND EXTRA TOTS. This is where making a Ulysses contract for party situations can come in handy. Doing the prep work to make sure you stay focused on your goals means that unexpected scenarios like this one won't derail your entire effort. You need a solid strategy in place in order to make sure you don't go off the rails and order things you won't feel great about later, or order things you're unsure you'd like and then wind up starving the rest of the evening.

Before you attend, assess how much wiggle room you have to make some menu-manipulating moves if you're heading out to a restaurant. Log on to the World Wide Web (that's what the kids call it, right?), and check out the menu. Pick out what you'd like to order, or which options look as though they can be modified in some type of way to make for a less heavy, less breaded/fried/cheese-filled/decadent meal. Know at least three appetizers and two entrées that you would feel great about, or think *could* be adjusted ever so slightly in a way that won't make you feel like a big ol' ~~pain in the ass~~ spoilsport to your colleagues or friends. If you do your menu homework, a wrinkle like the one I described above won't throw you off. F- those silly ~~sirens~~ tots! You're ordering shrimp cocktail to start, plus the roasted winter veggies with pistachios, and a slice of the wood-fired pizza you just ordered for the table. You're a *rock star*.

#protip

"For the table" can often be a trap that turns a measly eggroll into an all-you-can-eat buffet, simply because *Craig from the Kalamazoo office* ordered them "for the table." Offset this with a one-two punch of both your pregame snack (*you're not really hungry just yet!*) and setting the *objective* of enjoying *your* appetizer course *first*—before you get involved with the eggrolls. (Truth: I have a feeling you're not going to *want* 'em.)

Your Dining Out Ulysses contract starts with your best options no matter what, plus some ideas for where to start based on type of cuisine.

Dining Out Fallback Plans

When in Doubt: Skip the Grains

Before you flip over the proverbial dinner table on this one, hear me out. The reason why lots of "no-carb" and "low-carb" and "carb-free" and "keto" stuff has risen to the top is because of a common misconception about carbs that I feel we should really clear up right about now. I use the "skip the starch" concept as a jumping-off point with clients because it's my experience that, from a purely *behavioral* standpoint, it's a lot easier for people to not notice when they're grazing on the bread basket, having an extra bite of fried rice that was more like a cup, or an errant mu shu pancake, or simply going "overboard" before they even had a chance to feel full as a result of grain-based carbs in any meal. Let me give you a good example of this: Let's say you're ordering a side of sensible shrimp dumplings "for the table" and you have two (steamed dumplings hover around 100 calories a pop, so that's an extra 200). Tomorrow, you're at a dinner with other clients, and this one's at an Italian restaurant. There's a bread basket with some perfect-looking olive oil and balsamic just primed for the dipping, and you snack on one or two slices as the basket gets passed around the table (that's anywhere from 200 calories to upward of 400, depending on how much oil/butter and the type of bread/how many slices you have). The following eve, it's finally Friday and you're going out for some sushi and sake—you order a soup, a salad, and you split four rolls with a date.

All of these items—the dough on dumplings, the bread basket on the table, and the rice on said sushi roll are there on your plate as *vehicles* for you to eat the good stuff—Toro! Shrimp! Extra-virgin olive oil sourced from a protected piece of land in Tuscany! The end goal for you is to have achieved two things: feeling satisfied as a result of what you just consumed and feeling content that you ate something delicious you truly *enjoyed*. So that's why I often recommend to clients who dine out that they skip the grains as a part of their restaurant experience. The top-line rationale:

- You can get the flavor of the thing you wanted without having that little refined-grain vehicle as an addition.

- You're not skimping on carbs simply because you opted out of grains (starchy veggies, fruit, and legumes are still providing those—not to mention sauces, which are often sugar-containing without even tasting sweet).
- You can fill up from more nutrient-dense sources with more fiber (because, vegetables).
- You can feel solid about splitting a dessert.

Most importantly for understanding how to navigate dining out *for the rest of your life*: The starchy parts of any restaurant experience are often the part that you can make very easily yourself at *home*. If you say no as a blanket statement to starchy foods when you're out at a restaurant, the flip side is that you'll likely say yes to something more delicious and actually different from what you'd normally eat. If you're still hungry when you get home, you can top yourself off with something starchy—in a serving size that you have more control over. This is the simplest, most efficient way to cut back without feeling any form of deprivation at all. You're making a choice to eat toast for breakfast, or pizza when you're at a world-renowned pizza place. But more often than not, you did not make the choice to eat the equivalent of *four slices of toast* at a random business dinner on any given night of the week.

Remember, the primary goal is to get *you* to pay attention to the fact that you frequent specific restaurants for specific things: food specialties, cuisine staples, and perhaps even a cute bartender (in which case, go there for that, and snack before you leave!).

Saying "I'm not having bread at this meal" when you're at an establishment best known for their steak means that you're making the conscious choice to eat the things you want specifically from the places that are best for that food, flavor, and variety.

The Rule of Two

The rule of two is a strategy designed for any type of shared-meal scenario. It encourages you to think about which foods feel special to you in the context of a specific cuisine, place, travel destination, or restaurant, and makes regular restaurant eating easier to navigate because option overload is a recipe for snack-cidental eating instead of eating what you actually want and love.

In the rule of two, you'll pick two items that you love from two different parts of the menu that you might otherwise order if you were going balls to the wall on this meal. Think of it as your answer to the question "What would you want to eat at your last meal?" except more fun than thinking of just one answer. In this version, you get to choose a different "two" based on the type of cuisine or restaurant at which you're dining (*Lucky!*). Decide out of the three courses—apps, mains, and desserts, which *two* items you're going to have. These are more indulgent. Thinking about your level of frequency eating this cuisine, dining at this restaurant, or how often you'll be eating something *similar* should dictate which two items you opt in on. If you're going for steak tomorrow night with different clients, do you need the glazed spareribs or beef? You love dessert, but none of the ones on the menu speak to you—aren't you better off having a few bites of the key lime pie you *love* on Thursday?

The rule of two becomes the rule of "twice" when you are a person who dines out *every night of the week*. Then you'll pick two of these items, twice per week—because if every single meal involves loads of cooking oil, loads of booze, and loads of these types of options, then it's more than likely that you're either (a) sick of half of this stuff *anyway*, or (b) feeling like you already adopt a similar strategy as above, and aren't seeing any positive results from it on your weight or state of health, requiring us to pull the reins in just a smidge tighter.

It encourages you to get specific about the tastes and flavors you love, and maximizes the experience to leave you feeling satisfied—not stuffed. Case in point: You *love dumplings*. You've never even *met* a dumpling you didn't like! You're also A-OK to say that you *don't* want any of the rest of the stuff and choose two dumplings instead of one dumpling and one piece of beef that you don't care all that much about. The strategy helps you define what you like best, and enjoy a specialty at that *specific* place you're eating.

How much of the two items will you have, you ask?

USING TECH TO DETERMINE YOUR SERVING SIZE

FRIED FINGER FOOD = AN IPHONE CHARGER

Anything fried/doughy—like the tempura, the dumplings, or the fried mochi—opt for one (or one piece).

MEAT AND SEAFOOD OF ANY TYPE = AN IPHONE

Use your phone as a good baseline of how much of a sauced seafood or high-fat meat item to load onto your plate. A standard-size iPhone (5.5 inches) is roughly the size of the portion of meat or seafood you'd want to add to your plate. That said, you can eat more of versions made without loads of cream, sauce, butter, and breading—the more frills there are in the prep method, the closer you want to be to the iPhone-size serving. But poached, steamed, lightly sautéed? Feel free to increase the portion to a size more satisfying (like a cordless home phone of the early 2000s!).

FRIED/CHEESY/CREAMED VEGGIES, OR DESSERT "FOR THE TABLE" = YOUR DESKTOP COMPUTER MOUSE

ALL OTHER VEGGIES AND FRUIT OF ANY KIND = A FAX MACHINE! A PRINTER! YOUR DESKTOP MONITOR! A 3-D PRINTER! YOUR OFFICE *COPY MACHINE*!

In other words, these are always unlimited—even when *dressed*.

The rule of two also comes in handy at cocktail parties, buffets, and holiday meals in which you're not absolutely sold on *everything* being served at the meal and want to make a more nutritious choice, but hate the idea of having to "do without" shrimp tempura or dumplings.

Be conscious and pick smartly when it comes to the foods you want to eat at a given restaurant, and in a given time or place. Personally, my favorite place to eat ice cream is my couch, not an Asian fusion restaurant within a strip mall, but I leave these nuances to *you*.

Master of the Menu

There are often so many occasions when you're in a situation that unleashes a powerful dose of stress-provoking "What the f*ck do I eat *here*?" Here are my suggestions for the most challenging locales.

Dining Out

Appetizers

Absolutely anything raw bar at a place you trust: seafood, dollar oysters, tuna tartare, salmon or yellowtail crudo—these are high-grade options when ordered at most restaurants that can make you feel both filled up and satisfied enough to keep going while dining out. The beauty of all things raw bar is that they don't add sauce during the cook/prep phase. Ceviche, crudo, and tartare are alternatives that mean virtually the same thing and are prepared in basically the same way. Order an appetizer that's raw bar and a main that's heavy on the veggie, like roasted salmon with roasted summer squash salad with ricotta salata and cherry tomatoes! Or pasta primavera with a side of spinach sautéed in olive oil and garlic (ask for extra veggies and halve the pasta so you're getting a higher-volume meal for fewer calories). You won't feel like a stick-in-the-mud by ordering a salad with dressing on the side, but you're also not sitting down with a bucket of cream-cheese-stuffed crab wontons and calling it a night, *every night.*

Entrées

- Any fish order prepared "simply grilled," blackened, poached, sous vide, a la plancha, not in a sauce, + extra veggies
- Lean cuts of beef that include top round cuts, bottom round cuts, and sirloin steak
- Grilled or rotisserie poultry
- Veggies that are steamed, grilled, charred, blackened, sautéed, boiled, braised, raw, or roasted
- Starches you don't get anywhere/everywhere else

Desserts

- Petit fours: This is my favorite dessert absolutely anywhere because it's basically one of every dessert on the menu, without committing too early or wholeheartedly to something you don't actually love. Your average French macaron (a standard petit fours offering) is about 120 calories, give or take. Use that as a gauge for most petit fours plates (sure, it depends on the size of the petit four and whether or not it's cheesecake or a bite of berries, but stop overthinking it). That amount is roughly what you're drinking in a glass of wine or that Crown Royal on the rocks you're nursing. Thinking of it in those terms may help you make a choice between having another drink and having another petit four.

- Chocolates: Pick about three that look the best out of the bunch, and enjoy every delicious bite of those. Chocolate in *chunks, pieces, or caramel-filled heavenly bites* is an ideal dessert *choice* in any restaurant scenario because it's essentially its own contained entity. You won't be digging a fork into an endless block of chocolate unless your dinner is at Hershey HQ in Pennsylvania (*and even there, it would be slightly unique, no?*). There's a start point and an end point, and if you're at a good restaurant or at a place with great desserts, it gets even better. You can savor, enjoy, and move on to the next chocolate (or be done with it, since you're already so satisfied).

- Fondue (*seriously*): Secret power dessert is fondue—it comes with *fruit*! Which means that you're filling up with fiber-dipped chocolate! Dig in to as much fruit as your little heart desires, and keep that chocolate coating to an amount that's respectable enough to *not* drip all over the table and double as a sheet-mask for your face.

- Zabaglione: Another power dessert at Italian restaurants is zabaglione, made from whipped egg whites, sugar, milk, and happiness. It's almost always served with fresh berries, it serves as another vehicle to get you to eat more fruit, and it adds the perfect amount of indulgent flavor to something that might otherwise appear in your breakfast oatmeal. *Mangia!*

- Crema: Similar to zabaglione, crema is made without eggs and with heavy cream instead of milk. And while it may be slightly heavier than your lightweight, frothy zabaglione, it's still a means to an end in terms of getting you to eat more nutrient-dense fruit, making it a win all around.

#protip

If you're dining out every single day (we all have those crazy times), then let's go back to the rule of two for just a sec. If you're picking two nights of the week to opt in on the dessert course (versus skipping starch as a part of your "two" more indulgent items to choose when sharing), keep your eye on the prize in terms of what's really of the highest value to you.

The thing I really want you to remember here is this: You're not on a diet anymore, but every day is real life—no matter how busy or stressed you are, every decision you make contributes to the lifestyle you have. You have access to the information you need to know ahead of time whether or not the place you're dining on Friday will have the world's best pie, so the rest of your week may be without sad starches, bread baskets, and partially stale tortilla chips to really enjoy something that's *not worth missing (in all of its full-size glory!).*

On the flip side, there are some weeks where absolutely nothing is worth your attention, so you'll choose to have that treat at home or from something else you really enjoy *outside* of this meal. You have agency to make these choices by knowing what you're doing and where you'll be a whole lot of the time, especially in these business-related scenarios. Not all cheesecake, coconut cream, and fried chicken were created equal, so optimizing what you eat in the context of your month, week, and day leading up to said meal can help you feel more empowered about making choices that are right for *you* in any given scenario.

Brunch: A Buyer's Guide

Brunch, my conscientious readers, is a reminder to have a midday meal—let's not get confused simply because it's scheduled during a vast range of time slots on a given Saturday or Sunday. (*You can have it as early as 10 a.m.! Or you can have it as late as 4 p.m.! There are so many choices! Life is so confusing! Whatever, I'm getting cheese fries!*) But it's still based *on your schedule*, and presumably the schedule of the other people with whom you are "brunching." Meaning that your whole day of eating does not have to be mixed up by a meal that has a different consonant in front of it than it does during a given weekday. It, just like all else that you do in a given day or a given week, can be mapped out based on your schedule and your preferences. Let's have a look around the menu—then we'll get into your brunch-based weekend strategy.

Eggs + omelets (shakshuka, veggie omelet, cheese versus half-whites): These are always your go-to when you want to have a filling brunch that's also satisfying. Shakshuka = baked eggs with tomato sauce (often with cheese or spinach), which makes it the extra-ideal choice for getting in more fiber when you're tired of the ol' veggie omelet. Otherwise, both a regular omelet with lots of veggies and a half-white omelet that includes veggies AND cheese are your top choices. Eating the whole egg = the right amount of good-for-you fat that will fill you up and keep you from post-brunch noshing, but since brunch menus are often piling *on* the cheese in those eggs: Cut the amount of yolks in half so that you can savor the whole omelet without feeling exhausted and weighed down *after the fact.*

Veggies or fruit sides: All of the yes. Every time. Produce is always money well spent, so if you *don't* feel like a veggie or fruit side and you paid the errant few dollars for each or both: Cool. Take it home, and add it to breakfast later, or tomorrow, or add it to something else (e.g., add that spinach to a stir-fry).

Fries versus toast versus salad: You can *always* have the salad (see above point re: *vegetables*). But here's the deal: Choose the two slices of toast OR the fries or hash browns. Since servings of starchy stuff are always *large* when dining out, having both will be overkill (and all of us are susceptible to "picking" at whichever is leftover, even when we were satisfied by one or the other).

Bloody Mary versus mimosa: Bloodys are always a good go-to, but both hover between 100 and 150 calories, depending on (a) how much juice is in there and (b) how much booze is in there. If you're going for a mimosa: Order it "super light" or "with a drop of!" juice so that it's mostly champagne (or *just* champagne—and squeeze those orange slices from your fruit salad in there—when that option is available). But if you're not really for that, if it's a fresh, homemade, or tomato juice + spices prepped by the bartender: Go for the Bloody. Bloody Mary mix from a can is super high in sodium (it can pack up to 70 percent of your daily value!) so double-check with your waiter.

"Bottomless" brunch: If you're going for this, then you're better off going *sans* blood or mimosa, and going straight for the champagne that you're chasing with seltzer. See above re: that tip on orange slices! This will help you sip at a more sensible pace and cuts the hangover substantially by skipping the sugar from juice. Cut the starch from your meal in half to do this without going overboard—for example, one piece of toast or split the fries.

"Watching the game": Beer, wine, or any spirit on the rocks is about 120–150 calories, so stick with any and all of those for a better choice no matter where you are. And as for "light" beer—the calorie difference is negligible, but if you're having more than two or three, light might be the best option for you since this could easily tack on another 200 calories by halftime with the real deal).

Self-Sabotage at the Salad Bar?!?!

I know, I know: It seems like the salad bar should be layup for dining out, right? But the truth is, almost *anywhere* can be a layup for dining out when it's done right. Just the same, there are sneaky saboteurs to your energy level, weight-management progress, and dining out/menu-ordering confidence at the salad bar, too. Here are the top mistakes I see many of us make at salad bars and fast-casual establishments. Check in with yourself before your next order.

Your "fruit" is code for candy.

Think those cranberries are a savvy salad bar pick? They might be, but as is now very familiar, any dried fruit—be it raisins, cranberries, apricots, or whatever—is a source of added calories from sugar. Case in point: a ¼-cup serving of dried cranberries is about 100 calories, while a ¼ cup of seedless grapes is only 16! You're better off choosing the whole fruit option, be it sliced apples, orange slices, or those seedless grapes to add some sweetness to that lunch.

You're (a tad) confused about what a salad actually is.

The biggest salad bar mistake I see *all the time* is that a lot of us get confused about what the bulk of our salad should *actually* be, which is veggies! Instead, I'll often see clients adding scoops of fried wontons and tortilla crisps and croutons and breaded chicken with a beverage cup full of ranch, and there's barely a romaine leaf to be found in that plastic container! So, things to load up on: lettuce of any kind, cruciferous veggies (like cauliflower, brussels, and broccoli), eggplant, mushrooms, peppers, tomatoes, cucumbers, celery, snap peas, spinach, kale, artichokes, fennel, asparagus, and of course, marinated and grilled veggies. Next, choose one to two options from each section of the starch station (for a total of three): starchier veggies (like corn, sweet potato, or squash) and legumes (like lentils, chickpeas, beans, or peas). Add in your extra protein pick: chopped egg, chicken, turkey, shrimp, tuna, or beef, and top that veggie mountain with a scoop of cheese or guac. Sprinkle on nuts, seeds, and any salsa, spices, or hot sauce you like.

YOU ORDERED DRESSING ON THE SIDE

If you like what you put into the salad, there's often not much of a need for *dressing*. Here's why: Think of how some of the most delicious foods *become* dressing when they're in a salad otherwise: Salsa! Guacamole! Pico de gallo! Marinated, fermented, pickled veggies! Harissa! Sriracha! Hummus! And roasted/salted edamame! And my personal favorite: *a combo of cooked and raw veggies* (which is commonly available at places that do salads and "grain bowls")! If you're making this at home, it's even easier: You can smatter those veggies in the olive oil, garlic, spices, and hot peppers you've sautéed them in, so they'll dress the other raw veggies in the mix without additional labor. So my advice for "dressing on the side" is this:

- Dressing belongs outside of your salad if you know you like the ingredients within the bowl but you've never tried said dressing before and don't want to commit early. (*Great strategy there, Laurie!*)
- Dressing belongs outside of your salad if there are lots of dressings you'd like to try—order 'em all! Dab a little schmear on each different bite! (*You seem fun, Gary!*)
- Dressing belongs on the side if you're using it for something else (e.g., those aforementioned bar snacks).
- Dressing belongs on the side if you actually don't like salad at all and would much rather have veggies from soup, stew, sautés, or omelets, in which case, you might want to get off this salad line entirely, Linda.

Bottom line: If you're opting to bathe your salad in creamy ranch as a means to validate your choice of salad, you're not necessarily making a choice that helps you make satisfying food decisions on a consistent basis. (Some examples of that: bacon cheddar dressing; cheesy Parmesan dressing, and any dressing that rebrands itself as *aioli*. That's just *mayo—on your vegetables…perhaps it would taste better in the form of a sandwich?!*) And if you're ordering dressing on the side for reasons that are entirely elusive to you but have become a matter of habit, consider where you wind up on the satiety scale after a little bundle of shrubbery (aka garden greens). Are you starving? Are you full (*from sheer volume!*) at first, but completely famished in an hour or so? Because there's not that much energy density in that forest, so it's highly likely that as a direct result of this virtuous salad choice, you wind up eating the "For Sharing!" crackers on Diane's desk, leftover pizza crust from the afternoon staff meeting ("Just one bite!"), the contents of the snack mix at happy hour, and basically anything and everything left in your fridge at night, making this "healthy" concept null and void. Instead, opt for flavorful oils (like extra-virgin olive oil) with some real, wholesome, fiber-filled or protein-packed foods like avocado, cheese, hummus, or roasted/spiced nuts and seeds to give you the flavor you want combined with the lasting energy you'll need.

BYOB/F

So someone has invited you into their home for a meal, and you're stressed out about not being in control of your own ~~destiny~~ dinner. "Hey, man, just wanted to check what time you want us all there tonight. Need anything?" This text/call/email is a secret power move for when you're going to an event, party, or really anything hosted by someone else at their home or at any event space out of the home where there is not a set menu. (I think one might call that a *potluck*, no?) The point of this exercise is twofold: First, you get to be a good person. (*Proud of you, Billy!*) And second, you get to eat food that you might not actually get to eat if you were 100 percent *not* in control of a given situation. Here's another #protip somewhat off the record that I've used with clients frequently and in the following scenarios: Lying as a means of self-care. Yep, you read that correctly. You have my permission to "fib." It's a great way to tell everyone you're "intolerant" to a food or food group when you don't want to hurt anyone's feelings about the food being ~~inedible~~ not really your taste. I can't tell you how many clients I've *saved* from the perils of said scenario by using this tactic—not *because* the food you would eat otherwise at someone's home could make you sick, per se, or is really so inedible that you might as well be eating hockey gear. But fibbing with a "No worries, Marilyn! I'm actually intolerant to the [*insert ingredient name here* in Marilyn's homemade corn dogs]—but I brought this amazing Greek salad with shrimp with enough to share!" saves you from having one of those nights/days/events where you didn't like *most* of the things being served, and only enjoyed the taste of the chocolate cake/bread pudding/noodle pudding/croutons and wound up driving through McDonald's for a triple shake, triple fries, and triple Big Mac.

If bringing your own food seems like an extreme measure, listen up: There *are* plenty of people in the world with dietary restrictions—REAL

ONES—who have to do this all the time out of *necessity*. And you know what? So long as you are your polite and gracious self, absolutely *no one* cares. In fact, it's helpful—you made a side salad and saved Marilyn from having to do extra work, or feel guilty, weird, and inadequate that you pushed around your food the entire time and had nothing to eat otherwise, which as a host or hostess is a sh*tty feeling. So please, do everyone a favor and *lie* just a little bit now and again if you feel like it's more in line with your style of eating than Marilyn's. Cool?

Your Ulysses Contract for Any Occasion

Raise your hand if you've ever read (or heard of reading) a piece of content that states things like, "Put a note on your fridge before you go out saying, 'do not open!!!' when you get home to remind your drunk ass to not touch anything in the fridge!"

Everyone? Okay, *wonderful*.

That tactic is bogus for a few reasons. First of all, you can dress it up in a cute outfit with a bow, but that's a form of shaming *yourself*. Second, it's destructive and sets you up for failure. You just created a reminder of the fact that you might be hungry when you get home! So you know what your drunk ass is going to think about before bed? EATING. Before you go out for a rager where you're not sure what the food situation is going to be like, you eat a snack or a sneal, depending on your timing of (a) when you're leaving to go out, and (b) when you're (*REALISTICALLY, PEOPLE—NO JUDGMENT!*) coming home from said night out. Let's put it this way: If you're realistically coming home at 6 a.m., you've prepped ahead for breakfast!

Day-After Damage Control

Start your day with a cup of coffee. Caffeine is both a natural diuretic *and* an excellent source of antioxidants, which protect your cells from damage—so, as long as you are not caffeine-sensitive or chugging espresso all day, starting the day with your morning cup is a great way to kick off your bloat-defeating day.

Not much of a coffee drinker? Tea is also a natural diuretic, so choosing black or green tea can also help you hydrate while caffeinating. Herbal alternatives can have some diuretic properties (like licorice, or dandelion root), but teas touted as supplements aren't likely to deliver on the purported "health benefits" they're claiming (e.g., detox tea or fennel root). Bottom line: Drink whichever you like, but add milk of choice and skip sugary versions of coffee or tea lattes—especially of the frozen or whipped-cream variety. High-sugar foods, especially consumed on an empty stomach, can cause a bit of a water "rush" to your GI tract, which at best will make you feel slightly nauseated, and at worst will send you straight to the bathroom.

Next: Yes, you certainly need to drink plenty of water to help expedite the process of ridding your body of any sodium-induced water retention. But remember, that can come in the form of things you chew, too! Cucumbers, tomatoes, watermelon, asparagus, grapes, celery, artichokes, pineapple, cranberries—all of which contain diuretic properties that will also help you stay full due to their higher fiber, high water content.

Stick to your usual schedule, leaning heavily on the sneals (three sneals, three snacks—see chapter 4 for reference!). Keep in mind the combo of dehydration (keep drinking!), exhaustion (remember, your body thinks you want more carbs because it's on the hunt for serotonin!), and waking up with lower blood sugar (you're feeling sluggish and off-kilter).

Last: Consider adding extra sources of potassium, which serves as a nutritional counterbalance for sodium. Foods that are rich in potassium include leafy greens, most "orange" foods (oranges, sweet potatoes, carrots, melon), bananas, tomatoes, and cruciferous veggies—especially cauliflower.

Networking: It's More Than Just an Excuse to "Get Drinks"

Let's say you currently find yourself in a situation where you want to make plans but would rather not have to eat or drink. You have a number of options:

1. "I'm taking a break right now; let's go for a walk." Doesn't walking just solve everything? Seriously, though—warmer climates or summery weather makes this easier, so other alternatives for our frozen-weather friends:

2. "I need a manicure—can we do that instead of drinks tonight?"
3. "I am dying to see the Chihuly exhibit at the MoMA and was about to head there—come with!"
4. "Want to come to barre class/spin/dance/Pilates with me? I'm in the 6:30 class in Flatiron" (and follow up with a link in an email).
5. "I'm taking tonight off—rain check for Thursday?" Punt it. This has the added bonus of you setting your own boundaries for a change and getting out of doing something you don't feel like doing *tonight*.

9

Most of My Meals Are from a Take-Out Menu...(Okay, *All of Them* Are)

By the end of this chapter you will...

- have a guide to what to order *where*—based on cuisine;
- know how to make *any meal* lighter; and
- be able to use takeout plus foods you've got at home to make more nutritious options without adding extra time or stress to your day.

"Cheat Days" and Snack-cidents

"Do I get a cheat day?!" is a common question among victims of traditional diet culture, and it's typically associated with all food everywhere that can be ordered off a take-out menu. That's a tough confounder to navigate, since most of us are (a) eating lunch at our desks and (b) spending a lot of the day in front of a computer (with ready access to the *whole world of takeout out there*). To that end, "cheat days" and "takeout" are by no means synonymous! Let's start by clearing up this "cheat" language for a moment: My answer to this question is usually delivered with one word:

"NOPE!"

Here's the thing about cheat days: They aren't a real *thing*! That's because every meal is the first meal of the rest of your life; this isn't a diet, so there's nothing to "cheat" on!

Truth: Through the lens of your new mind-set, you eat the foods you want to eat once you know your "why" as it relates to what you're ordering. That means you're not ordering deep-fried cookies and hot dogs "by accident." (I commonly refer to this type of eating as a "snack-cident," because in case it wasn't already clear, I'm a sucker for a good pun.)

Eating what you want also means that you must pay attention to why you want what you want when you want it. How do you determine why you want to eat something you've previously restricted? Well, you know that one already!

1. Check in with your willpower sh*t starters. Are you exhausted? Hydrated? Did your physical activity level change?
2. Recall some Right-Now Rules, and see if any (or all) apply: Did you eat breakfast today and was it filling enough? Have you eaten regular meals and snacks (and were they satisfying)?
3. Do you really want two slices of pound cake, or did you just "hold the bread!" on your sandwich and want something chewy and spongy? If yes, then you have two choices:
   - Pick something else that will crush this hankering because it's similar to the consistency of what you want but is really replacing what you missed in the meal before. Good examples of this: a piece of toast with fancy-flavored nut butter (e.g., Muscle Butter in Glazed Donut, Wild Friends in Cinnamon Raisin, Buff Butter in Birthday Cake, The Big Spoon in Chai, Julie's Real Cashew Butter in Vanilla Cinnamon).
   - Choose the pound cake, because you really do just want pound cake even though you might be satisfied by another option, but pound cake sounds amazing right now! You eat it, you love it, and you move on with your day.

It's completely true that a day of eating anything/everything is (relatively) harmless in the scheme of things (weight loss or maintenance and your general health), but for some, dedicating the *whole day* to eating whatever you want can spiral into a No Baked Good Left Behind campaign in your neighborhood, or double-fisting cheeseburgers from the couch— all of which has the opposite effect. But the other biological hazard of the "cheat day" is that it's really tough to get back on track eating regularly because you start out *too full* the next day, and it's also a mental and emotional roadblock for many of us. That's why consciousness is key: Dedicating a day to calling yourself the human Cookie Monster can have the effect of putting a "cheat" cycle on loop: You're stuffed and feel like garbage, so you don't make it to your morning workout; you skip breakfast and lunch and have powerful heartburn (and a whole lot of generalized fog), until you can finally eat dinner, which, because you're now hungry enough to eat a whole pizza, is "Two pepperoni pies and a side of garlic bread, please!" (Right?!)

In the same way that you now consider 80:20 as your mostly attainable-yet-somewhat-aspirational ratio for trying new health-focused things, the real, advanced-level goal is to be so consistent with all of your regular habits that you lose this language altogether. This happens simply by making conscious indulgences a part of your everyday life (and therefore, removing their power over you and your food choices entirely!). But since that can be a challenge for every single one of us, doing a little bit of prep for yourself can at least make these indulgences more frequent (rather than being labeled "cheating" and therefore off-limits!). You can choose to eat meals, snacks, and desserts that may not make it into your repertoire daily, but do it as a direct action following a choice you made for yourself rather than an accident.

That way of thinking (and eating!) can help you stay on track long-term and sets you up to make healthful choices that include the foods you love—from any menu, anywhere and everywhere.

What to Know Before You Go (or Order In)

These are the top mistakes I see when choosing from a take-out menu that throw so many of us *off* our game! Think about these before you Seamless:

Be Wary of a Promotional "Deal"

I don't mean to wax philosophical here, but I do believe it was a great thinker of our time who said, "You won't save money on a lunch deal today if you have to buy new pants tomorrow." (Okay, maybe it was just me who said that.) But the advice is (hopefully!) just as sound: If it means spending a little extra (just a few bucks—not $20!) to make a more nutritious and satisfying choice (ordering two apps to make a whole meal, being choosy about which sides you want with which main, adding a veggie soup to your order, or adding the $1 each for avocado), then it may be worth your while to spend now to feel pretty awesome in a few hours, not to mention better health in the long run!

This is especially true if it's something that you know will have a greater impact than, say, getting the three-for-one special of sushi rolls (FYI: that's *three* cups of rice!) when you could have had a miso soup, a salad, a roll, and a few pieces of sushi and a rice-less handroll (which is always a markup, but real talk: If you're ordering sushi to begin with, you already know it's not the McDonald's dollar menu! So your expectations are already in line with paying a little bit more than you would if you ordered sushi every single meal, every single day. So you have my permission: Treat yourself).

Do NOT Contract FNSS

Have you ever ordered a burger "without the bun" because you thought it was healthier, but then ended up feeling a little disappointed after? I hear you. If you've skipped a "group" of macronutrients (protein, fats, and fiber-rich carbs) entirely—like ordering a protein-less pasta dish, having a veggies-only salad, or eating a sad little grilled chicken breast at your desk—then you are well aware of takeout-induced full-but-not-satisfied syndrome. FNSS happens when we try to cut calories from the wrong places and wind up feeling a variety of symptoms that could be anything from peckish to raging at the office vending machine: "HAND OVER THE DORITOS AND NO ONE GETS HURT."

Just because you ate *enough* sad desk-chicken doesn't mean that you'll be satisfied for too long without the help of a little whole-grain bread and sliced avocado.

Ordering When You're Hungry Means You're Too Late

Place your order when you're at a 5–6 on the satiety scale, and make sure you're (a) hydrated and (b) getting your snack on regularly that day—every three to four hours, of course. That's key to staving off the graze, because takeout can often be delayed, which means another hour or so will go by until the doorbell actually rings. Avoid the trap by making sure you've got a mid-morning snack on days you know you're ordering in. Even something small, like a piece of fruit stashed in your desk drawer, will add a little fiber (and help hydration!) so that you won't gulp down the pizza pie upon arrival.

TOP TAKE-OUT HACKS

If you're opting for takeout and looking to make more nutritious choices, some general tips:

- Double up on veggies no matter what you're ordering. Burrito today? Extra sautéed veg. Chinese? You'll have a side of the garlic green beans. Pizza? You'll have a slice of the veggie and start with a salad, please.
- Order your sandwich on 100% whole-grain bread instead of a wrap, roll, or "flatbread," which often have extra oil added during baking.
- Nix sour cream or cheese-based spreads, and double up on veggies no matter what you're ordering.
- Check out the kids' menu—there are some great options on that list that are the right price and size.

ORDERING A SANDWICH = A POWER (TAKE-OUT LUNCH) MOVE

Sandwiches are the BEST, right? They're also one of the most nutritionally complete items you can eat because they combine a whole lot of fiber with protein and fat—and you know what we call that now, right? An FNSS-CRUSHER! But I often see clients who find sandwiches to be a little bit tough to wrap their minds around because there's so much loaded *crap* that comes in store-bought versions, and there's lots of confusion about the bread. So, here's your sandwich-making strategy 101.

Make Veggies the Star of the Show

Start by piling on as much as you want of those dark leafy greens (higher in B vitamins and minerals than traditional butter lettuce), and add your favorite veggie toppers like sliced tomato, cucumber, onion, mushrooms, sprouts, zucchini, peppers, and eggplant. Use any leftovers for a side salad and dress with lemon juice or balsamic vinegar to taste.

Pick an All-Star Bread

Choose 100 percent whole-grain options and at least 3 grams of fiber per serving. Hint: The first words on the ingredients list should be "whole grain," *not* "enriched wheat flour," a common code for white bread in disguise!

Choose Your Lean Protein

Choose 4 ounces (about 4 slices) skinless chicken or turkey breast if you're going in on meat. Roast beef is great, too, and about the same from a nutritional POV, but it can be a higher-sodium option. To keep sodium at bay, look for lower-sodium brands at the deli counter or choose rotisserie options; you could also just opt out of the meat altogether and choose seafood, like canned tuna or salmon. Also, who says eggs can't get involved in this midday delight?! Scramble two whole and two egg whites with lots o' veg and you've got yourself an omelet with toast—but also a sandwich. LOVE. IT.

Add Some Fat

Mayo's A-OK. It's higher in fat than other condiments—about 2 tablespoons of the white stuff is about 100 calories versus 60 calories in the same amount of hummus—but if it's your bag, then add it based on a schedule (e.g., twice a week if you're eating sandwiches daily). Otherwise, opt for a flavorful spread of 2 tablespoons of hummus, or a third of an avocado, because these provide some fiber and nutritional benefits sneaking in in the form of antioxidants (extra!). Next, add a slice of mozzarella, cheddar, pepper jack—whatever you love—for extra deliciousness and protein (1 ounce = about 8 g protein, which makes this whole meal more satisfying). Know that options like soft feta or goat are often a lower-calorie "cost" but are intense in flavor, so add to sammies with a lighter hand if you're aiming not to overpower the other ingredients in there.

Give It a Kick

Season your sandwich with 2 tablespoons of spicy Dijon mustard, salsa, or roasted veggie tapenades (like red pepper), which boost flavor without racking up calories.

Menu Showdown: A Dietitian's Journey Through All Your Favorite Cuisines

Do you ever get to the end of a workday, week, or even particularly stressful weekend, and think to yourself, "*Ugh, I just want someone to tell me what to do!!!!*" Same. That's why I did all of this background work for you, so that you don't have to plan ahead or think too much about any given dining experience once the only thing that stands between you and Netflix is a meal.

Asian Fusion

Strong starters: The primary ingredient to watch out for in Chinese/Asian fusion food is sodium. Stay hydrated before, during, and after your meal and choose foods with high water content like (you guessed it) vegetables. Steer away from fried options—words like *tempura* and *crispy*. *Steam* is a great word here.

    Entrées: Choose steamed items as your mains, like chicken and broccoli, shrimp and broccoli, and so on, and opt for a super-flavorful sautéed veggie dish to add in there: String beans in garlic sauce, sautéed "sweet and sour" broccoli, and the ilk—you can't go wrong on this one unless it's breaded and deep-fried. When the meal arrives, you've got a mostly steamed option with a satisfying flavor-bomb in the form of *vegetables*.

What to skip: The fried rice, the battered protein, and pot stickers stuffed with cream are not your best bets. Also high in sodium and saturated fat (and a whole lot of starchy, low-fiber, sleep-inducing carbs) are rice noodles—all the refined carbohydrate that won't fill you up with fiber. Look out for high-sodium entrées that can have your entire day's worth of salt in one sitting. You want to steer clear of "combo" meals, surf 'n' turf, anything that will have gigantic portions unless you're ordering them for your whole table to enjoy (and therefore, you're only having an iPhone-size-worth of it, and the rest of your meal is lots o' veg—of course!). Noodles: These dishes are really high in salt and calories and you are getting a lot of starch. A better option are the udon noodle lunch bowls—just add on some veg.

@ HOME DIY: Do the noodle bowl your way by controlling the sodium and adding extra veggies from what you've got at home (steamed or sautéed in sesame oil with Asian-inspired seasoning staples, like ginger, garlic, umami paste) that you'll par-cook (not all the way through!) and add to the batch bubbling on the stove. You can add items like veggie noodles, or some others that lend themselves to use in soups: Shirataki noodles (which stay their same slippery consistency whether they're in soup or not!) and Palmini noodles (which are canned and made from hearts of palm—they retain their pasta-like texture while cooking). Of course, you can always opt for traditional buckwheat or soba noodles; these veggie swaps add more fiber and leave you room to lighten up the meal and fit some protein in there, too, such as grilled (instead of fried) poultry, seafood, beef, or bean (like tofu or edamame). Choose a "low" or "less sodium" broth base, and season as you like once you've combined all the parts together.

Another at home DIY you already know by now: Veggie "fried" rice, which works best sautéed and a teensy bit charred with sesame oil, scallions, ginger, umami paste, and—regardless of all else that goes in there—sriracha (if you like it spicy) and a fried egg that you'll add into the pan and scramble into the mix.

Sushi

Strong starters: Seaweed salad, mixed greens, *oshitashi* (boiled spinach salad with roasted sesame and soy sauce) or *nasu* (grilled or broiled eggplant with miso) are all lower-calorie picks. Other great go-tos: Miso, mushroom, or seafood soup that's broth-based—the combo of liquid plus umami flavor helps you fill up before you dig into your main course. Split edamame with a pal to load up on 8 grams fiber, 11 grams protein, and important minerals like magnesium and iron.

How you roll: The key is to stick to *one* six- to eight-piece roll per meal (surprising stat: There's anywhere from ½ to 1 cup of rice per roll!) and keep it simple: Choose brown-rice rolls that combine fish (salmon, shrimp, tuna, yellowtail, etc.), veggies, and avocado. The satisfaction trifecta of filling fiber, protein, and healthy fat is optimal for staving off cravings and keeping you satisfied. If one roll just won't cut it: Add a Naruto roll (which swaps rice and seaweed for cucumber wraps), or my favorite trick: Rice-less hand rolls, which add a sandwich-like quality to your order (think: Shrimp and avocado wrapped in seaweed paper). Plain ol' sashimi is great too—add up to three pieces to your order.

What to skip: Frills, like cream cheese, spicy mayo, dumplings, and spring rolls, or anything deep-fried. Since they're often tough to spot on a menu, look for words like *creamy, crispy, crusted, crunchy, spicy,* and *tempura,* or skip the specialty rolls altogether—they're often high-calorie (from sugar-sweetened sauces and saturated fat) for very little satiety benefit.

@ HOME DIY: ANYTHING "CRUSTED," "FRITTI," "CRUNCHY," OR "CRISPY"

Anything you might otherwise eat battered and fried at a restaurant can, in fact, be consumed by sautéing it and flavoring with the condiments or sauces you like. Shrimp is a great one because adding a little bit of citrus juice or marmalade helps flavor "stick," plus you're heating up that skillet with oil and butter, which lends a flavorful hand. Add garlic and onion powder, chili flakes, paprika (or any seasoning you like) and add crunch at the end as desired (e.g., toasted coconut chips for coconut shrimp; chickpea crust like Watusee Foods' Panko Chickpea Breading for more savory versions).

Mexican

Strong starters: Salad, soup, or salsa, and ceviche, *por favor*! Choose lightened-up *empezadas* with tons of veggies, plus avocado, shrimp, chicken, or beans, and a sprinkling of cotija cheese (it's a lighter, less powerful cousin of feta).

Be a smart tamale: Order tacos or fajitas with double veggies and a side of *frijoles* (black beans) instead of rice—peppers, tomatoes, mushrooms, and greens are often cuisine staples. Fill 'em with protein that's prepped *a la plancha* or *a la griglia* (in a pan or on the grill). These are always great picks: Fish or seafood, chicken, hanger steak, or vegetarian options, and opt for the corn tortillas (dig into three per meal)—they're lower in calories than wheat versions. Can't imagine Mexican without the guac? Neither can I. Order the more decadent dips (sour cream, refried beans in sugary sauces, etc.) with your main course instead of as a starter; you'll be more likely to keep portions in check once you've *already* had an app. Top your platter with a heaping tablespoon each of your favorite(s), like guacamole and cheese. As for salsa—go *HARD on those spicy sauces!* Salsa is amazing because it has virtually zero calories (okay, more like 20–40 per serving, per type—but still!) and is loaded with tomatoes, aka *more produce* (and what's not to love about that?!).

Order the chips after you've had your appetizer and in between the app and the main course. The word "bottomless" comes to mind, which is used to describe both the chips themselves (*$3/bottomless chips at happy hour!*) and often a feeling in our stomachs that we couldn't possibly ever *stop eating these damn corn chips*, bringing on distorted thoughts like, "What if I literally never see a corn chip again and I said no to this bottomless basket?!?!?!" But if you go in on a half-full stomach, you're far more likely to have a few and move on. And if you're really keen on sticking with my advice here, I'd urge you to skip the order entirely 80 percent of the time if you eat out or order in from Mexican restos often. Because while it may seem like you'll never see these bottomless, partially stale, fiber-free, deep-fried shells of their former vegetable selves (*yes, corn started as a vegetable, too!*), you *will* see them again when you dine at this restaurant tomorrow and the next day, and you'll certainly see them in their more satisfying (less bottomless) form at the grocery store, where you can check that the first ingredient says, "100 percent stone-ground corn" or even better, "beans," and feel satisfied from a more nutritious nosh that'll quell the "bottomless" feeling. As for plantain chips, these are similar in nutritional value to corn chips, depending on where you're getting them, but having one or two of the grilled version is a great choice to swap for other starches, like rice or tortillas, since they deliver potassium (a counterbalancing mineral to all of that salt) and fiber and help you fill up.

#protip

If you do like spicy foods, hot sauce, or are generally a self-proclaimed salsa aficionado (condiment, not music . . . but hey! *You seem fun, too, Carol!*), order one of each type of salsa that's offered, and use that in place of dressings, dips, or even as their own ingredient in veggie-heavy salads or sautés. These add fiber (especially in a heaping scoop of a heartier type of salsa—one that's made from corn and beans!) and provide a *ton* of flavor, without sending you into a sour cream–induced food coma.

What to skip: Frozen margs, bottomless tostadas, gorditas, carnitas, burritos, tamales, quesadillas. They're all calorie bombs from added sugar, saturated fat, or refined starches (which rack up calories quickly!). Other toppings to skip: Queso, crema, and chorizo, which are common at Mexican restaurants. Last, double-check the meal prep: Items like fish tacos often seem like the healthier pick, but look for words like *Baja* or *battered*, which are just nicer names for "deep-fried"; you can usually ask for them to be grilled instead.

Pizza

Strong starters: Pizza joints almost *always* have a salad option, but switch it up by ordering the *antipasto*, so long as there're loads of veggies involved on that plate. While it's best known for its high-in-fat processed meats and various different types of heavenly cheese, adding grilled, marinated veggies can bring both flavor and fiber to the ho-hum salad you'd order otherwise. Pack that plate high with flavorful additions like olives, peppers, anchovies, artichokes, and roasted peppers, which add rich flavor and a special element to your meal that helps you savor each bite. If you're planning on definitely diving into the pie once it arrives: Choose either your favorite cheese or your favorite type of cured meat, and stick to two thin slices of each (or two slices of one type, if you're not as into one of those). (Personally, I'd urge you to go "cheese" instead of "meat" on this one because, let's face it: If you're going to a restaurant known for pizza, they're more likely to make damn sure that's some excellent cheese and tomato sauce they've got on hand, right?!). An even better option: Order the antipasto with other appetizers that provide leaner protein, like grilled chicken, grilled shrimp, or grilled calamari (basically anything grilled will do it!) and have one of these to yourself if you're planning on just having a small slice or opting out of the pizza entirely (you can make your meal more filling by adding a legume-based app, too, like chickpeas or lentil salad, offered in most Mediterranean cuisine).

Top it off: Don't skimp on toppings to "save" calories—you'll only wind up craving the leftovers later on! Instead, fill up on fiber by loading your pie with unlimited veggies, add lean protein like grilled chicken (or a sunny-side-up egg, if you're going the artisanal route!) and throw in some sides: Garlicky sautéed spinach and broccoli or eggplant in marinara are flavor-packed picks that add tons of volume to your order. Take *that*, second slice!

What to skip: Any vegetable that's been held hostage by the deep fryer, and the "*Extra* trifecta": Extra cheese (e.g., "four cheese" slices, mozzarella sticks), extra dough (garlic knots, bread), and extra meat (sausage, bacon, and ham).

@ HOME DIY: Swap out traditional crust (or sad frozen pizza you've had in the freezer since President Reagan was in office) and opt for a better base: cauliflower. You can buy these crusts at the supermarket and use as directed. Load these up with extra deliciousness by sautéing some veggies to go on top of that cheese and add protein as you like. You can even add little "pockets" of part-skim cottage cheese while the pie is in the oven for more protein without loading on calories from higher-fat meats you'd get if you'd ordered in the pie.

MISTAKE NOT TO MAKE: ORDERING SALAD WHEN YOU WANT PIZZA!

No matter how much parm you grate atop your Caesar, there's no amount of cheese that turns lettuce into deep-dish. The same is true for cheeseburgers, tuna melts, and, er, *grilled cheese sandwiches (because cheese is pretty much the star of that show, no?!)*. That said, if you're a little unsure *WTF you're really in the mood for*: Start with cheese as part of your snack or sneal before you head out to lunch or dinner (midmorning string cheese; 1 ounce of cheese with a piece of fruit in the afternoon, or Parmesan crisps), which will help you discern if it's the flavor or the full-on food you want right now.

Italian and Pasta

Strong starters: In Italy, portions are not universally "smaller," but there's an emphasis on vegetables as a major part of each course of each meal, so that when you eat pasta and other heavier courses, you wind up eating smaller portions of things that rack up calories faster, rather than doing the exact opposite. With that in mind: Starters will likely be similar to those on your pizza menu—opt for either a big salad to share or a soup that's veggie based if you're planning on a meat, chicken, or fish entrée as your main. Other great calls on an Italian food menu: Carpaccio, en cartuccio, or branzino, which is basically on every Italian menu in the United States and is also deliciously paired well with just about every wine, vegetable, and client on planet Earth.

    Secondi *on fleek*: Opt for pasta dishes with at least two veggies already in the dish, and ask for another veggie that sounds appetizing to you on the side. (Sautéed spinach with garlic and olive oil anyone?) Toss that in with your pasta, and mangia away. Sounds like a whole lot of veggies, no? Well, my cogent readers: IT IS! Because that's what pasta is supposed to be like! So when you wind up eating it the real way, you still get the flavor and the deliciousness of the ingredients *within that dish*, but you also have the benefit of cutting way back on the amount of starchy carbs you're eating (that aren't satiety-promoting) while actually eating *more food* than you might have otherwise. And you're not "sacrificing" anything, either. You're simply adding fiber to an otherwise *lower fiber* dish. Look at you! You're basically a chef!

What to skip: Again, any deep-fried version of an unassuming protein or vegetable source (Zucchini! Calamari! Meatballs!) or anything with the description of "fritti." (Yes, folks, that's *fried* in Italiano!). I'd also recommend skipping here anything you could make at home. Reminder: There's no point in doing something that feels "indulgent" to you if you don't actually enjoy it all that much!

@ HOME DIY: Try using a legume-based pasta at home to make any pasta palooza more satisfying. These are about 21 grams of protein and 18 grams of fiber per serving, which means that not only are you about to feel extremely full, but also there is little *physical space in your gastrointestinal tract* to feel remotely deprived or as though you didn't get the "humongous bowl of pasta." Make sure you're dining on these with some extra H_2O for drinking. Fiber is best digested, absorbed, and utilized by having water both to help it *move through your GI tract* and to help it absorb biochemical waste that turns into cholesterol, so give your intestines a helping hand by drinking a full 8–16 ounces with said dinner. Now, relax, eat pasta, and prepare for a bowel obstruction (*JUST KIDDING!*). But seriously—I'm oversharing the specifics on this information because something that my clients have never gotten "used to" is the fact that when you have a lot more fiber in a type of food that normally doesn't contain *as much* fiber, you wind up getting real full, real quick. So pay attention to how full you're really feeling as you eat; don't assume that you're going to need to eat as much as you would if it was regular old semolina noodles, capisce?

Bar and BBQ

Appetizers: Veggie-based soups, like tomato basil, chicken and vegetable, or chili; chicken, beef, or shrimp skewers of any kind; and any other option that so happens to be grilled instead of deep-fried.

Mains: Any grilled meat or seafood item, like "grilled chicken with _____."

What to skip: This is a tough one, because most bar food exists as its own treat (Wings! Nachos! Bacon cheeseburger! Wings! Cheese fries! Wings! Spinach artichoke dip! Buffalo ranch dip! And WINGS!!! Did I mention wings?!). So here's where timing and frequency are key: Unless you find yourself at the local Brother Jimmy's *more than one day per week*, the stuff to *skip* is the stuff you'd otherwise order in the name of "health." Just enjoy the damn food for what it is (i.e., foods that aren't *everyday foods*), and plan the rest of your week around today's indulgences. So skip salads, if it was a virtuosity order versus an actual desire to go light for any *other* reason. I mean, *seriously: YOU AND I BOTH KNOW THAT WE'RE NOT HERE TO HAVE A HOUSE SALAD, PENELOPE.* And for the love of all things delicious, please *do not order the fruit plate at a bar*, unless you're into that—in which case, do you. (A glass of wine can, in theory, double as the fruit plate, too, if you want it badly enough...)

If you *do* order from a bar menu more often (two or more times per week), think of it this way: Which aspect of bar food do you like the *most*? Is it the dip? Is it the wings? Is it really just about the beer and not about the food at all? Consider your favorite aspect of the meal, *do add in those extra veggies* from wherever you can find 'em, and build your meal around *that*. For example, let's take those wings. Order the wings, have three or four hearty pieces of those babies, and pack the rest of that meal with veggies you love. Or, maybe you don't care all that much about the wings, but you *love that bleu cheese dip!* Ask for more than just three sticks of celery with your wings. (Carrots! Broccoli! Tomatoes! Asparagus!) If the bar is offering a salad on their menu, then they do in fact have these in stock—you can ask for extra! Choose the crudités as the swap for your base instead of the fried corn chips, pita chips, or cheesy fries.

@ **HOME DIY BAR FOOD:** Fried chicken in all of its forms (wings, nuggets, tenders, and baskets): Some people live for wings. Other people eat wings (or tenders, or nuggets...but especially those nuggets if you have kids!) because they're simply *there* all the time. If you fall into the category of someone who lives for chicken wings, then by all means, decide when and where you're going to have said wings, and go with it (using the knowledge gleaned from the rest of this book already). But if you fall into the latter category, you're eating a lot of battered breading that you could easily skip by maximizing flavor with a sensible *dry rub*! Buffalo, buffalo ranch, spicy ranch, and spicy bleu cheese rubs are a savior here for when you'd like to eat winged goodness, but would also like your pants to button all the way. Have grilled or rotisserie chicken with said rub, and dip poultry into premade dressing, dip, and hot sauce/sriracha/Tabasco. Some great brands for doing just this include the following:

- Frontera dry rubs, spices, mixes, and salsa flavoring
- True Lemon dry rubs and spices, Primal Palate Spice Blends, Trader Joe's Spice Blends
- Mrs. Dash dry rubs and spices
- Tabasco dry rub
- McCormick dry rub
- Hidden Valley spice rubs and dressing "rub"

When you *are* dining out at a place where the only option is chicken wings and you are going to be eating there every single night for a month or two, take note: Chickens existed in the world long before the deep fryer was even invented! And that's great news for you, because it means that you can, in fact, order any grilled chicken item and add some sauce to that situation so that they still maximize the part of the wing experience most everyone loves. (Buffalo sauce! Ranch dressing! Bleu cheese dip! Spicy hot sauce happiness!)

Indian

Strong starters: The fare from the East is great for vegetarians and everyone who loves a burst of many flavors and an onslaught of spices. The spices used all have marvelous health benefits, too, plus beans and lentils are cuisine staples, making it easy to mix and match items. These are a perfect pick for choosing a lighter menu item while still getting fiber and protein (not to mention magnesium, potassium, and antioxidants!).

Curry without worry: For mains, think anything tandoori, or masala, and all kinds of kebabs all the time. There are some hidden gems in Indian fare, since the cuisine is heavy on veggies and spices, often making it lower in sodium and higher in fiber than other forms of takeout. That's not a universal truth, however: Opt for items with dal (lentils, turmeric, ginger, black pepper), which will pack upward of 8 grams of fiber per ½-cup serving. Other great veggie sides: chana masala (made from chickpeas, spices, and coriander), veggie curry, eggplant curry (baingan bharta), and any item swapping tomato and tomato sauce as the base instead of coconut milk. You can't go wrong with any lean protein cooked in a tandoori oven, nor can you overdo it on "tikka" (so long as you're eating those veggies!).

Say "nah" to naan: Try some delicious roti, which is the whole-grain version of the fluffy, pillowy traditional naan bread (often slathered in butter and oil, driving up the calorie content but without any satiety-boosting nutrient combo (since it's lower in protein and fiber). Have a slice of the roti with lots o' dips, which are mostly made from fruit or veggies as their base—mango chutney, tomato sambal, and cucumber raita are all great—and follow the "bottomless chips" guideline of ordering roti between your app and your main in order to stave off a "bottomless bread" situation.

Coffee House

Skip

- Whipped toppings, which at Starbucks add about 150 calories just from sugar and fat (so while delicious, they're not going to make you feel full or caffeinated—the two main goals of going to Starbucks in the first place!).
- Tea lattes are also sneaky at Starbucks, because the tea powder used to make the lattes contains added sugar, as well as the sweetener or syrup that's added to them—and if you order almond, coconut, or soy milk, those are *also* sneakier sources of added sugar as compared to regular cow's milk. For example: A nonfat grande chai latte provides 43 grams of sugar, while one made with coconut milk is 39 grams of sugar. The sugar found in regular milk is naturally occurring, so even though it's technically "higher," it's still less from an added source (just a touch sneaky, right?!). Regardless, my best tip for ordering a tea latte at Starbucks is to ask for a regular brewed chai tea of any size, and ask for a side of hot milk (of your choosing). That way, you're skipping the sugary powders and/or syrup, getting some sweetness from the milk, and you can add a little non-nutritive sweetener or a dash of regular sugar, and cinnamon/nutmeg/cocoa powder/vanilla powder to your heart's content from the condiments bar.
- Frozen bevs are delicious, but unless you're specifically going to Starbucks for a dessert in Frappuccino form, skip 'em (have a milkshake,

right? The line is shorter at the diner!). These are often just sugar, ice, and milk with a little bit of coffee (the fancier ones have whipped cream and loads of other syrups and sugary flavors). The light versions of these bevs are okay, too, but since there's ice and milk added in, you may be getting less actual caffeine than you'd like, so choose these for flavor and less so for any nutritive benefit that you might want from a cup of joe.

- Your best bet for teas and lemonade is to order them unsweetened. While a grande (white tea, green tea, or passion fruit tea with lemonade) is only about 90 calories, it's 22 grams of added sugar (which, you now know, is 5½ teaspoons in a serving). Plus, while sugary drinks can taste refreshing, you may notice you're *still thirsty* once you're at the bottom. That's because sweet drinks can have the effect of making you thirstier, so you're better off spending that cash on a venti unsweetened version and sweetening on your own.

- Ones to avoid: Any of the juices, juice-based drinks, or smoothies. These are mostly just concentrated sources of added sugar, which can make you thirstier and won't fill you up or keep you satisfied. Opt for whole fruit and drink unsweetened bevs so you can get the real bang for your buck when you head to Starbucks!

Okay to Have

- **Whole-milk cappuccino.** Anytime, anywhere, a regular cappuccino can be a great order—it's indulgent enough to feel like a treat, but it won't set you back a whole lot in terms of calories—a tall cap made with whole milk at Starbucks is only 110! Since cappuccinos are made with foamed milk, you'll still get the jolt from the espresso and creaminess from the milk—but ordering these nonfat is a little unnecessary since they're so low-cal to begin with! Add your own flavor with cocoa powder, cinnamon, and vanilla, and you've got a delicious morning bev with 6 g of protein and about 75 mg caffeine (more if you add extra shots!).

- **Nonfat/low-fat café misto.** A misto made with low-fat or nonfat milk is a great choice. Since it's made from coffee instead of espresso, you're getting more coffee and less milk than you would from a latte, making it an optimal choice for mornings when you just need some extra caffeine! Plus, when you use less milk, you're automatically cutting back on calories, so it's a better bet if you're looking to cut back without skimping on your morning coffee beverage. You can also order these with a pump of sugar-free syrup if you're looking for some extra flavor!

- **Iced or hot tea (black, green, rotating unsweetened seasonal flavors).** These are virtually calorie-free and super hydrating, and they'll be lighter on the caffeine if and when you're looking for it. Herbal teas are just 15 mg of caffeine, while caffeinated black and green teas will still pack around 45 mg per grande cup (for a grande iced coffee, you're getting around 165 mg—up to 200 mg if you opt for cold brew).

- **Skinny vanilla latte/skinny mocha latte.** Since these are made with a sugar substitute, they're fine for a treat—especially since they'll also pack up to 15 g of protein for a 16 ounce (grande)! Lattes made with nonfat milk provide naturally occurring sugar instead of the added type, plus have the benefit of packing protein, which can help you fill up. Since they taste sweet, they're better for those times you just want a bit of a fancier bev without overdoing it on calories (160 calories for a grande skinny mocha; 130 calories for a grande skinny vanilla). An underrated, delicious pick during the colder months: Skinny Peppermint Mocha (you're welcome!). That little bit of mint flavor forces you to sip slower and make that deliciousness last longer.

- **Iced or hot cold brew.** Fans of cold brew coffee love the creaminess and smooth taste. And since these tend to be naturally sweeter due to the brewing process (room temp for a longer period of time than traditional pour-over, at a high temp), you'll be less inclined to add sugar or sweeteners. Plus, cold brew can be higher in caffeine content than traditional brew, making it a better "bang for your buck" if you're only stopping at Starbucks once a day!

10

I'm on the Road So Much That I Barely Know Which Time Zone I'm In, Much Less What to Eat Once I Arrive!

After this chapter, you will...

- strategize the right food-related Ulysses contract for any vacation or business travel;
- have a fallback, go-to strategy for food-related travel scenarios in which you have limited menu control;
- perfect the art of the packing list;
- learn and practice smart hydration habits to offset time zone changes and jet lag; and
- build better-for-you habits into your already-in-place travel routines.

By now you know that healthier eating habits are formed in the minutiae of your day to day. And while it's incredibly annoying to hear "everything adds up!" or "any exercise counts!" the truth is that doing as much as you can, whenever you can, will become ritualistic over time and lead to your healthiest, happiest self.

When traveling, the greatest challenge to get over—for absolutely *every* client I've seen—is that feeling of helplessness that comes from being in different surroundings. So whether you're navigating a time change or just a pit stop, this chapter is about giving you strategies for keeping goal oriented regardless of where you are or whom you're with. I'll give you a guide to beating the perils of time zone changes and how to navigate when you're stuck with a travel delay (I'll give you specific snack ideas for what to eat depending on the length of your delay, and how to handle it when you're just going to post up at the bar and drink until *your* wheels are up). Last, we'll discuss how traveling and feeling bloated inevitably seem to go hand in hand, and we'll walk through what to do before (to avoid it) and during (to minimize it). And remember: I know this stuff is tricky, but it puts you in control. The more often you put these habits into practice, the more likely they are to stick.

#protip

Your goals shouldn't change when you're on the road; sticking with the same set of priorities for your food, exercise, and sleep is the best way to avoid the travel hangover that makes so many people wish they could have a vacation after their vacation!

Wait, but Where Are You Going?!

The crucial component is thinking about your packing list and travel necessities as *inclusive of your health-related needs.* It's not demanding to tell conference planners that you can't have red meat every night, or to check that they'll have plenty of water, or to ask for a schedule ahead of time so that you can figure out if you'll have time for a visit to the hotel gym if those are the things that you need to feel your best—and especially if those are the things that make you an active, engaged, focused, and generally proactive person to *be around*, much less do business with! If you're thinking, *"Great, thanks, Jackie; now I have to figure out what I'm going to wear for a week AND think about what I'm going to eat? No thanks,"* then you're really in for a treat—because doing it once means you'll know how to do this going forward, and it's going to be super simple and fun! And yay! *You're going away!* (Even if you didn't think you wanted to accompany Bob from accounting to Tuscaloosa this week! Honestly, he needs *you*.)

Packing List = Travel Strategy Ally (TSA)

The major difference between eating on the road for a work-related reason and eating on the road for a vacation purpose is that in the latter, your time is more often *your own*, meaning that you can determine when and what you eat with (sometimes!) a little more flexibility. But for work, if you're attending a conference, traveling with colleagues, meeting with clients or potential clients, or flying solo with the big boss, you may not always feel like you've got freedom to do what you need to do—and the same goes for what you eat. That's why your packing list is so important—it helps you feel prepared and in control, no matter who's running the itinerary.

Stress-induced eating, as we've already covered, can take many forms and can come from many sources. Food is often tied to feelings, such as loneliness, homesickness, fear, or just generalized anxiety about a presentation. This can make it hard to focus on your ultimate goals when you're on the road. So when it comes to nutritious items that you know make you feel better and can prevent you from feeling "off" when you travel—that's when it's time to bring some in-case-of-emergency snacks for your bag of toiletries.

In general, your travel-related "tools" for better, healthier travel habits will include plenty of snacks for the road.

Let's pretend for a moment that travel of all kinds (but especially work travel…) is a marathon. (*Those who are reading this line in real time from the Delta lounge and accidentally shouting, "preach!" are about to make things awkward with your boss, btw.*) You'd need sustenance and fuel on which to keep going so that you can actually make it to the end. A similar physiological process happens when we travel, though it's not to the same extent. Often, we wind up depleting mental and emotional energy because of a consistent need to make conversation, other people who get all up in our personal space, travel delays and security lines that have us ~~crying to TSA agents about missing our flights~~ wondering if humans could possibly move any slower than they are right now, etc. You need consistent fuel in order to keep going, but in this scenario, there's no depletion of glycogen storage. But for the most part, staying on schedule with meals, snacks, and proper hydration is key to helping you avoid making choices you'll later regret. Here are my go-tos.

Cereal

Cereals, especially hot ones, are the easiest thing to put in a carry-on, especially ones that come in those single-serving packs or mini-cups (although those can take up a bit more space). The beauty of having something like this on hand in your carry-on is that you can split up breakfast by having part of it in your room no matter where you are. Oats are also an easy base for basically anything available to you at a hotel or during any travel experience. What you're looking for is something that can stand as a meal all on its own.

Look for brands that have protein and fiber in great supply and be as low in added sugar as possible: About 300 calories, 6+ grams of protein and fiber, and aim for 8 grams or less of added sugar. The latter should be more like 80–120 calories of plain, instant oats in prepackaged, sealed little packs. These are ones you'd combine with some hot water and nut butter/nuts/ fruit on the ground if you were looking for something more substantial, or if you just wanted a nice little bedtime cereal snack with milk. These should be a mix of plain and slightly sweetened versions, because these smaller portions are a little bit sad/taste and look like gruel when totally flavorless. Look for ones that have "6 grams of added sugar or less per serving" (9 g is ideally your max per cup) and have at least 4–5 grams of protein and fiber per packet.

Beyond the Cereal

If you don't want to eat sad gruel in your room by yourself, that's A-OK! You're not Oliver Twist asking for *more* (*though it may be how you feel when you receive your bimonthly paycheck*). The sole purpose of having a dry, easy-to-pack, single-serving whole grain on hand is so that when you're stuck in a pickle (which in this case looks a lot like having the option of bacon-wrapped-bacon or deep-fried butter for sustenance), you have something physically with you that you know is nutritious, easy to eat with many different types of *other* foods (including hot water or hot milk, or overnight with milk in your mini-fridge), and won't spoil for at least a year. Another option is a BYO whole-grain, fiber-filled cracker, which makes it easy to turn literally anything into a sandwich with a lot of fiber and fewer refined carbs (the kind that are all too easy to eat, rack up quickly in calories, but, most importantly, put you right to sleep in the middle of a dim, over-air-conditioned conference room). Here are a few great choices:

- Flackers
- GG Scandinavian Bran Crispbread
- Kashi 7 Grain Sea Salt Crackers
- Wasa Crisp n Light Rye Crackers
- Wasa Whole Grain Crispbread
- Dr. Kracker Seedlander Crisps

#protip

If or when a sit-down breakfast isn't a mandatory part of your travel plan, you can often partake in a breakfast buffet by grabbing eggs, lots o' fruit, and whatever protein and produce you love (Veggies! Cheese! Smoked salmon! *OMG marinated mushrooms?! I love this hotel!*) Bring them up to your room while you get ready for the day.

Bars

Bars are key for travel because they're portable, and buying the right ones isn't as difficult as it used to be. Look for those that have a real fruit, vegetable, whole grain, nut, seed, or nut butter as the first ingredient. There are three types that all have uses when packing—kind of like clothing *layers*!

- Fruit-based (100–150 calories): KIND Pressed, KIND pressed + chocolate; That's it! Bars; Lärabar Fruit + Nuts/Lärabar Minis. Use these as a light nosh between meals.
- Nut- and fruit-based: RX Bars, Nature Valley Protein, KIND Protein, KIND Nuts and Spices; Lärabar. Use these when you're nearing the 3- to 4-hour mark but won't have access to a more substantive snack for at least an hour or two.
- Whole-grain-based: Clif Bar Crunch, Kashi Granola Crunch, Nature Valley Peanut Butter; KIND Squares/Popped. Use these as a breakfast base or sneal base (with a pack of nut butter).

Fruit, Nuts, and Seeds

These are some serious travel essentials, because no matter where you are in the world, unsweetened dried fruit is going to provide you with fiber and crucial antioxidants that help you fill up and protect your immune system. Nuts and seeds (and iterations of each) are packed with some fiber but will also give you plant-based protein and healthy fat—meaning that a combo of these foods is the epitome of a "satiety trifecta." These types of snacks travel well, are easily packed, minimize spoilage (and bugs/animals lurking at your destination), are nutritious, and also help make *other things more nutritious and tasty*!

Some solutions:

- Unsweetened dried fruit: Peeled Snacks; Nuts.com packs + mixes; Sahale packs and mixes; Mavuno Harvest dried mango, jackfruit, pineapple, or mixes; Sunsweet unsweetened dried snacks (apricots, prunes, apples, pears); Montmorency unsweetened dried cherries
- Nuts, seeds, legumes: Eda-Zen Edamame packs; SuperSeedz 1-ounce packs; Saffron Road Crunchy Chickpea Snacks; Biena Snacks 1.5-ounce snack packs; Watusee Foods chickpeatos; Manitoba harvest toasted hemp seeds
- Nut butter and seed butter: Soom Tahini, Wild Friends, Nutso, Barney Butter, Justin's, Justin's Banana Chips + Almond Butter; Nutso Seed Butter; Sunbutter Cups

---

SPEED ROUND: MAKING A MEAL OUT OF (AIRPLANE) SNACKS

An assortment of snacks can also replace less nutritious burger-and-fries or sandwiches stuffed with processed meats. Try combos like these:

I Love Sweets! Can I Make a Meal Out of Sweet Snacks?

1 Sargento Balanced Break + 1 piece of fruit + Justin's PB; 1 pack Sahale/Planter's honey roasted peanuts (1.5 ounces) + hard-boiled egg (2) + frozen/fresh berries

Savory Only, Please!

Yumami snack pack (chips + hummus) + 1 part-skim string cheese + Blue Diamond Almonds 100-calorie packs; Stuff'd vine leaves + Peeled Snacks dried pineapple + 1 ounce Wonderful Pistachios packs

All in One Sneal

GoPicnic premade to-go lunch packs; Peanut Butter & Co. to-go lunch packs; Horizon Organic Good & Go lunch packs = all premade options that serve as healthier versions of old-fashioned lunchboxes!

I Want a Sandwich!

GG/Wasa/Mary's Gone Crackers/Flackers (whichever high-fiber cracker you like—your pick) + Barney Butter Almond Butter + 1 apple, pear, or banana (sliced) + 1 crudité cup with a side dip + 1 Babybel cheese

Okay, but What About *Snack-Fast*?

Or snack breakfast: hard-boiled eggs + fruit salad + crackers to go (2) + 2 tablespoons peanut butter + 16 ounces nonfat milk with cinnamon and cocoa.

Sweets to Go

If you like sweets, read carefully: Keep dessert *in your room*. Yes, really! Having a little treat to look forward to that's on hand at the end of the night is crucial for sanity, but it's also crucial for you making intentional, informed, better-for-you choices no matter where you are on the *planet*!

Let's use the example of the dreaded conference dinner for a moment. Let's say you ate well, made solid choices, but maybe you didn't fully achieve a perfect six or seven postdinner on the FNSS scale. Dessert comes, and you've just been through the marathon of all presentation days (I mean, *nonstop! Barely a bathroom break!*) and you're f*cking *exhausted*. Even though you still have work to do, you want something sweet because you made all of the food choices you wanted to make today, so you dive into some exceptionally mediocre conference cheesecake that was clearly frozen and is now thawing and has strawberry sauce that tastes just a touch like plastic drizzled on top. You eat the whole darn thing and then some of Bob's, but are then even more full and less satisfied than you had been before.

The onslaught of feelings that develops from this spans a full range, from totally harmless and easily solved with a little water and calcium carbonate (*that's a chewable Tums, for curious minds*) to full-on self-loathing accompanied by a subsequent shame spiral that leads you to feel like you should definitely give up now before your presentation has even started— and before you've even put your final touches on slide 17!

So how do we avoid the potential pitfall that is conference cheesecake and the spiral down it may lead us? Treat yourself! Order dessert in the room. It (a) gives you a little something to look forward to, and (b) allows you to indulge with something you *actually like eating* (not plastic conference cheesecake), in a place you actually like eating it (not at a conference dinner table). It looks like this:

- A bag of Hershey's Kisses; leave yourself 9, and put the rest away.
- Mini-candies (3 snack-size Snickers; 1 pack of peanut M&M's; 1 regular-size Three Musketeers bar; 4 random chocolate minis of any kind, etc.).
- Chocolate-covered nuts (½–1 ounce if it's real chocolate; a heartier 1– 1.5 ounces if it's something chocolate dusted, like Skinny Dippers).
- Ice cream bar or cup that you can buy in packs of four and leave in your room's freezer or one you eat right away.
- A decadent idea: Order off of the room service menu and enjoy every bite with your feet up. That way, you can be choosier about your own personal taste (and therefore, more satisfied) and get a higher-quality item (like petit fours, chocolate, fondue, or zabaglione, or berries with whipped cream, etc.). Your homework: Do this dirty work ahead of time to find out what's *actually on that menu* before you arrive at the hotel so that you can plan ahead.

#protip

"Make Peace with Food"

This "step" in the practice of intuitive eating asks you to keep previously "forbidden foods" around you and within your midst more often. The idea is that the more you have these things, the less desirable they become. So while I'm *not* advocating putting yourself into a situation where you feel out of control, if you know for sure that you can't possibly keep a bag of Kisses at bedside and have a few without inevitably eating the whole bag, I am asking you to consider the fact that the more exposure you have to the things you've previously restricted, the less power those things have over you. You *will* eventually get to the point where you just don't care if your hotel room is above Willy Wonka's Chocolate Factory if you commit to putting this strategy into practice regularly. A good time to try on this new practice could very well be in a new environment, when you're a little bit out of your routine and your comfort zone. Travel is a chance to get away from your usual habits, so use this contained period of time to try something different and see how you feel. If it's too much for you based on where you're at right now, toss it and go.

Moving On the Go

You're in a conference, in meetings, or even just flying somewhere for a meeting. Or you're on vacation with your family, loving life by the pool and reading all of the books ~~and maybe this one for the third time~~. No matter where you are, a part of your new healthier-habit practice includes *moving your tushy regularly*.

(You didn't think I was going to let you go to Cancún without *sneakers, did you?!*)

Often I have clients who are simply in the habit of *not working out when they're not at home*, and that's just silly as a principle *alone*. This doesn't mean you're "going to the gym" when you're on the road; it means that you are able to walk places or get something else done while *physically moving*, in order to serve the purpose of achieving better mental, physical, and emotional health. I had a client we'll call Tim the Traveler. Tim went *weekly* to a massive hotel in Boston, where he consulted for his work during the week. He *packed only* work clothes for these trips—not comfy shoes, not workout clothes. Honestly, I'm not even sure he packed socks—and he worked *all day*. Adding something new to his regular routine wasn't really on the brain at 10 p.m. on a Wednesday. But he did talk to his family on the phone for an hour every night while he was there, four out of seven days of the week. So I suggested that he do his call home on his headphones and go for a stroll around the hotel property. He *loved* it! Well—he realized he loved it the week after his first travel-trial, when he had no appropriate footwear for said occasion (*I believe blood and Band-Aids were involved*). But moving forward, the footwear was the game changer. Once he got back from long dinners and put those sneaks on for his nightly stroll, Tim was on that phone for *at least* an hour—he didn't have to add anything to his already long to-do list, but he really enjoyed talking to his family while he was exploring a new area for the very first time.

Tim wound up losing an extra five pounds more than his initial goal between when he started his walkabouts and his return to my office three months later. He used his iPhone to track his steps, and those nights had him clocking over 10,000 for the day. That's not to say he wasn't making *plenty of other tangible shifts* in his personal health management, but the major turning point was that Tim no longer felt like his travel schedule was putting him on hold for where he needed to be weight- and health-wise. Once he realized how he could do more in a way that didn't feel like adding extra responsibilities, he started making changes to his daily routines regardless of where he was. He kept up his walking routine while in Boston, even venturing outside of the hotel sometimes, and when he was in New York the rest of the week, he loved walking with his family in Central Park.

The Three T's: Timing, Type, and Tools—the Travel Edition!

Let's put our strategizing to good use and take this show on the road: Enter your three T's: type of travel, timing of your activities, and the tools you'll need in order to execute. Go, team!

Travel Type: Absolutely any travel of any kind, anywhere in the world
Timing: All day, every day
Tools: Unsweetened nonalcoholic beverages (and some choice foods you already love!)

Hydration is a word that sounds a bit like a snooze but is your single greatest ally when you're traveling. Granted, if you're reading this still: You already know that staying hydrated is key, but when alcohol is literally *on the agenda* for your company-wide retreat or your beach vacation, this is your number one priority in terms of your health and to make sure you're eating consistently, feeling (at least somewhat) energized, and able to tell the difference between when you're actually hungry and when you're slightly peckish (but really just thirsty).

Regardless of whether or not you're partaking every night, getting in this habit (even if you do *nothing else!*) sets you up for making better choices and for feeling better overall throughout your trip.

- Wake up and drink: 16 ounces first thing in the morning, before you get out of bed.
- Have water with you at *all times*. ATTN: READERS: This is NOT a drill! You need water (or some type of beverage!) *on your person* no matter where you are and what you're doing! Altitude from air travel dehydrates you; running through train stations dehydrates you; different cuisines and different destinations may have saltier items on set menus that your body may not be used to—*this makes you dehydrated*! You need a 16-ounce bottle or travel mug with you at all times, but you should also know that ho-hum water isn't your only method for achieving this goal. Try sparkling water; flavored sparkling water (without sugar or a sugar substitute); unsweetened iced tea; or unsweetened coffee (meaning, without sugar—you can add your own

sweetener or non-nutritive sweetener, or drink it on its own—just no prebottled sugary drinks, which will just make you thirstier!). Make your travel goal an extra 16–32 ounces (2–4 cups) more than what you're (now!) used to drinking. Add more if you need it, but unless you've been given specific directions by a physician to *not* drink a little extra H_2O: Cheers!

HYDRATION BEYOND THE GLASS

If you're experiencing that REM-cycle-disrupting pain that lasts under a minute but feels like someone is taking a saw to your calf, there's a good chance you are...you guessed it! DEHYDRATED. But it's not *just* about the liquids, in this case. It's highly likely that you're suffering a little electrolyte imbalance that's a direct result of *not* consuming enough sodium, potassium, calcium, or magnesium, or is specific to just one. This is a common one if you're walking frequently in hot weather. Here are some extras to add to your diet if this sounds like you:

- Magnesium: Leafy greens, nuts and seeds, legumes, avocado, bananas, dried fruit, chocolate
- Calcium: Dairy products, leafy greens, fatty fish, seafood of all kinds, almonds, soybeans
- Potassium: Tomatoes, potatoes, oranges, bananas (and all other fruits and veggies)
- Sodium: Every-f*cking-where

Travel Type: Conferences, presentations, conventions, and meetings
Timing: Determined by the "agenda"
Tools:

Sound-free snacks: You know what's terribly disruptive when you're giving a presentation? Some dude in the front row crinkling a granola bar wrapper that's seemingly impossible to open and crunching it audibly when you're *just trying to get through annual growth metrics on slide 4.* On the other hand, you probably don't want to *be* that person either, so it's best you plan ahead with some sound-free snack items you can take with you to avoid going past three to four hours without a nosh:

- Unsweetened dried fruit (Peeled, Bare, Dang, Mavuno Harvest)
- Nut butter packs and tahini spread (Justin's, Wild Friends, Barney Butter, Artisana, Peanut Butter & Co., Soom Tahini)
- Literally any soft cheese—but get that thing out of the wrapper before the lights dim/Todd from the Chicago office gets this show on the road (Sargento Snack Bites; Polly-O String Cheese, Arla Cheese Snacks)
- Leftover fruit plate from breakfast (*Who knew you could find a use for that filler-fruit, cantaloupe?! It goes so nicely with your cheese snack and it's basically the quietest snack you can find—win!*)
- Olives or vac-packed veggies (Love Olives, Gaea Olives)
- ½ PB&J sandwich

Eating to stay awake: Skip starch—grains, potatoes, and the bread basket—at lunch. Here's why: The amino acid tryptophan is taken up more readily by receptors in your brain when your pancreas secretes insulin, the hormone that takes up glucose, and deposits them in your cells—leaving what's leftover (those amino acids) to float happily through your blood–brain barrier, where it's converted to serotonin and subsequently melatonin (the hormone that makes you *pass out in the middle of the most important part of the session*. But also, *poor YOU!*). It's the secretion of insulin that triggers this cascade of hormone responses and makes you feel like the only thing that could possibly save you from a REM cycle is a Jessie Spano–on–caffeine–pills dose of caffeine. It's a simple strategy to apply "skipping the starch" for general weight loss, and it's an even better bet to skip it at lunch in this (or any other) setting where you're tasked with being seated for a prolonged period in an airless room in the middle of the day.

Travel Type: Work, but with bottle service
Timing: Late nights, later-than-usual mornings, mostly no sleep
Tools: Attention anyone, everywhere working in finance—this is you!

You've spent all day in a conference room, though you're not even sure if it actually *was daylight* today because you've been inside for what feels like at least twenty-four hours. Now you're going out to blow off all of that steam on the company dime. Great! But can you really do this nonstop every night and not gain weight? Well, no...but also, *yes*! Here's what you do:

Choose your "party" nights: Real talk—no one can have one of those nights where you're *literally* (and figuratively) leaving it *all* on the dance floor, every single time you leave your hotel room. But in the spirit of also *not* becoming the group spoilsport, how can you actually do this and feel comfortable doing so?

- Alternate every drink you have with a glass of sparkling water. This doubles, of course, as a drink for the moments in which you need it to (a sensible garnish is really the only apparent difference between a club soda and a vodka soda—a maraschino cherry is kinda fun, too!). With this in mind, however: Many of us are rolling our eyes thinking, *"Yeah, right!"* so if that's you (*I see you, Mike!*), then think of it this way: When it comes to hydration, just *do more* than where you're at normally (which for you, buddy, is the middle of the Sahara without a Nalgene).

- If there's a dinner with alcohol involved, stick to wine, beer, and champagne (sorry, Bob, no sangria tonight for me!) OR...

- Nurse a top-shelf spirit, neat or on the rocks. Slow and steady wins the race on this one. The top-shelf pick (do your research ahead of time!) makes you look like a badass but puts you in the driver's seat of how much you actually take in (versus drinking champagne or vodka soda or any other mixed drink all night that can be easily topped off). You sip at whatever pace works for *you*, but choosing this route prolongs what you drink (since it's *physically more difficult to just swig the whole thing down in one gulp*) and is also about as strong as you can possibly get, meaning that you're still partying with the best of 'em but not necessarily taking in more calories than you would otherwise.

- When you get back to the room: Drink another 16 ounces of H_2O and keep the time frame contained so that you're going to bed thirty minutes to an hour from when you arrive back in the room, whenever this is a feasible option. That decreases the time you have to expel unnecessary emotional energy by scrolling social media and reading email and eliminates a tear through your travel snacks/minibar after your night out.

Use the Agenda to Reframe a Habit

I want you to get comfortable with the idea of reframing the health-focused things that you like to do in the context of a travel setting. For example: You want to run every morning of the conference. Realistically: Is that feasible with the agenda? No. But there's a late start on Wednesday, and an extra-long lunch on Friday, and Thursday there's a *three-hour gap* between the last speech and dinner. You can run during all of those times! Just as building new habits at home starts with your schedule, having travel routines and rituals can be positive, too—but if you travel often, you'll have to get comfortable with the idea that these may change, *every single time* you leave home. For example: If you're keen on breaking a sweat every day and your current job regularly lands you in LA for work, then maybe you *love* hiking Runyon Canyon in the mornings before you start your day. (Awesome!) But can you realistically *hike a canyon* in Des Moines, Iowa? Not so much. (*It's pretty flat, amirite, Iowans?!*) Similarly, you may *always* order from the omelet station when you're in Dallas—*"Add all of the veggies! A slice of pepper jack! Extra hot sauce, please!"*—but now that you're in Philly? There's no breakfast included (and your company does *not* want you ordering a la carte from the menu!).

If you can't do the travel-related things you did last year, last week, or even yesterday, it does not mean they can't *inform* what you're doing now and provide you with information to get you to take action when you're on the road. You love a Runyon Canyon hike? Go on a run and explore Des Moines! Or go to the gym! Or use one of those fitness streaming services you started playing around with before your flight yesterday! No veggie omelet this morning? NO problem! Starbucks has eggs! Or the CVS has hard-boiled eggs in a two-pack! Go grab those, and use what you've packed to make for a hearty morning meal that's both protein-packed and full of produce.

(*Reframing is so FUN!*)

Eliminate Time Gaps

What if I don't like the gym in the hotel? What if there's no running path? What if all of the machines are taken? What if this group yoga class is totally embarrassing and I can't do any of it and all of my coworkers (who are in way better shape than I am) are there? These are all examples of fears that have been shared with me by previous clients who have just a teensy bit of anxiety about trying new habits on the road. So do yourself a favor this way: If you're planning to break a sweat in the morning, get those gym clothes out, put sneakers and socks on the side of the bed, have your headphones/devices charged up and ready to roll—whatever you need to get out the door, do it for yourself ahead of time so that there's no *time* to question whether or not you want to go when your alarm goes off—you need to go now, or skip it, because one more minute and you're going to miss the morning session.

(*Bye! Have fun! Wear sunscreen!*)

Travel Type: Vacation!
Timing: All on you!
Tools:

The beauty of having this type of unlimited free time is that your schedule is all your own—hooray! Kind of, but sometimes this type of scenario can create a crushing feeling of debilitating anxiety because you don't even know where to start and there's so much damn relaxing to do and what *do you even do first*?! Well, you have your own pseudo-vacation style, and I'm not going to tell you what to do with this time! But I can suggest that if you're planning on exercising, you do so early in the morning (and by early in the morning, I mean whenever you wake up—so if that's noon, then *awesome!*). The reason for this is directly linked to hydration, which is extra hard in a tropical locale where there's lots of beverages to be had and lots *more* lying down to do.

All-you-can-eat buffet: Use the rule of two, but with a more specific strategy. This one can be *super tricky*, especially because most of us have this nagging, pit-in-the-stomach feeling that we cannot possibly NOT EAT EVERYTHING at an all-you-can-eat or all-inclusive buffet.

Start with a BIG plate of fruit—go hard here, and treat the omelet station as if it really is your best friend. In general, if you picture your plate (or meal on the whole) the way this book is (basically *always*) telling you to: 50 percent or more should be from vegetables and fruit. In this case, get yourself a big bowl of fruit because treat yourself, you're on vacation! And luxuriate in the fact that you don't have anywhere to be and can eat your fruit in peace with a foamy cappuccino and—you guessed it—a glass of water.

Before you leave the table, do a little satiety scale assessment: Do I feel good enough on both ends of that equation to leave right now? If yes, grab a little treat to go (and you can have it later on or after dinner!). If you're full but not satisfied—you know you're probably missing an egg or two, or missing a slice of toast or a piece of fruit or BOTH. So go back, get what you know you'll need in the fiber family or the protein family, and if you feel so inclined, add a little healthy fat in the form of peanut butter, cheese, smoked salmon (or other available smoked fish) or a spread (like tahini, hummus, yogurt, etc.) to use for a topping, snack, or part of a sneal later on.

#protip

Reminder about all-you-can-eat *anything*: This is a boundary bully, dressed up in a resort lobby. Your boundaries are still *your boundaries*! Just because you're here on vacation doesn't mean you have to go *all in on pineapple upside-down cake before 8 a.m.!* "All you can eat" is marketing for *food on holiday!* So, remember: You do you. You're still going to pay for breakfast regardless, so you might as well enjoy it *full circle*—how it tastes and how fueled up you feel to carry on with the rest of your day.

Beach drinks: The idea behind day-drinking on the beach is to have some *fun, right?!* Consider ordering a glass of wine and a bottle of sparkling water, and be friendly enough at that swim-up bar to ask for as many garnishes as your little heart desires. Pineapple! *Maraschino cherry!* Citrus rinds! Whatever it is that makes a beach drink feel fancy to you, get yours.

Why rosé all day can (really!) be your mantra: One glass of wine is about 120–150 calories (for a good and generous pour). If you've got a liter of sparkling water that you consistently add in to the vino (*Maybe even ice? Is that gauche? Who cares! You're on adult spring break!*), you're accomplishing a whole bunch of goals all in one: Hydrating while you also imbibe; physically filling up a little so that, even though you're drinking, you're still in touch with where you actually are on the satiety scale, offsetting any kind of hangover symptoms that could last you until tomorrow (and avoiding FNSS because you're still eating like you would otherwise).

What not to have: A daiquiri, a piña colada, anything that's served in a punch bowl or a coconut half, anything with the suffix "punch" or "iced tea" (when you and I both know that's not *just* "honey" in there) and anything with—wait for it—juice. Here's why: The sugar that's coming from those mixers spikes blood sugar, while alcohol itself *lowers* blood sugar (and blood pressure). The result? A massive hangover, and a f*ckload of non-nutritive calories that you'd never normally consume on an average Thursday.

Other good options/wine alternatives: White wine, champagne, anything "with soda" (club, not tonic!), or any type of day-drinking that includes a bottle-service scenario where there's some juices that are brought out with limes, citrus, and—you bet—garnishes. Ask for extra water/ sparkling water/spa water, and pick the real fruit over the concentrated version (maybe even ask for a cocktail umbrella, too!). This will get you fiber, antioxidants, and some extra H_2O you'd miss from *just* sugary (hangover) juice.

Bikini Body: The Myth That Keeps on Giving

The day that "flat belly foods" become a thing is the day that pigs fly. It's not actually, physically possible to "spot train" any one area of your body with food, nor is it 100 percent true that you can universally spot train *period*. Weight loss of any kind helps to move fat stores for breakdown and energy use from *everywhere* in your body, but if you store more fat in your midsection, then weight loss will help move the needle. But as you now know, all myths are the leftover remnants of a diet-driven lifestyle, and there's no place for that here. With this in mind, remember that bloating is different from the concept of "belly paunch," "pudge," "puff," and whatever else type of insult you may have hurled at yourself in the past. Bloat comes from a few different places, but when you're traveling, it's most often linked to three culprits:

1. Sedentary time at 30K feet⟶ altitude's effect on your circulation
2. Changes in hydration and food-adjustment period
3. Constipation

Here's the background of what's happening when you feel puffy, blown-up like a blueberry, and uncomfortably *full*: You're experiencing shifts in fluid and electrolytes (sodium, potassium, calcium, magnesium) in and out of your blood cells, which can occur at this (*totally innocuous and normal!*) degree as a side effect of water retention (dehydration, excess salt, and altitude). The result? Vasoconstriction, tightening of your blood vessels, and a virtual *standstill* of your intestinal tract (*or at least it can feel that way, right?!*). So whether you're accidentally doubling your salt intake with one of those sodium-laden in-flight meals, or you're on the move so much that you're not getting your usual 8 glasses of water a day, travel-bloat is a common occurrence. How can you combat it? Glad you asked.

1. **Fill up on "fresh."** When it comes to bloat, sodium is public enemy number one. While limiting sodium from the saltshaker may help, the sneakiest sources of sodium come from packaged foods and processed goods, like white bread, bagels, and baked goods; canned soups and sauces; condiments, cereals, and even some beverages (hint: just say no to the midflight Bloody Mary!).

2. **Use prepacked produce:** Ready Pac, Rockit Apples; Cup o' Cherries; Cal-Organic Farms; Sun Basket "Flavor Bursts"; Dill-It-Yourself; Dandy Celery + the Peanut Butter & Co. Snack Packs = easy ways to add produce when you're on the go.

3. **Choose bloat-busting brew.** Another win for your morning cup of joe: Caffeinated coffee is a natural stimulant, the effects of which enhance peristalsis to keep things moving through your digestive tract. Since having regular bowel movements is key to a tighter-looking tummy, drinking about 8–16 ounces of java at the same time every day (the earlier, the better if you're caffeine-sensitive!) can help keep you on schedule—it takes about 30 minutes to work its way through your system. Remember: Sugary espresso sips (think caramel lattes, frozen drinks, and whipped-cream toppers) can lead to weight gain, so build a weight-friendly, health-promoting beverage by skipping fancy flavorings and choosing a nonfat café au lait or misto; compared to lattes, coffee-based drinks are lower calorie, since they leave less room for milk.

4. **Dine on dairy products.** Add a cup of low-fat dairy, like milk, a stick of part-skim mozzarella, or ½ cup of low-sodium cottage cheese to breakfast, and you may have a belly-busting win: While some studies

have suggested that diets high in calcium may be linked to lower body weight, results from a 2014 study published in the *American Journal of Clinical Nutrition* suggest that calcium-containing foods may reduce waist circumference in those genetically predisposed to carrying weight in their midsection. Plus, the potassium found in dairy products can have counterbalancing effects on bloat-inducing salt.

- **Try it:** Plain Greek yogurt with sliced banana, which helps stave off tummy troubles by promoting the growth of "friendly" bacteria in your gut—an important aspect of staying immune to travel-induced illness.

5. **Go nuts.** According to a 2015 study published in the *Journal of the American Heart Association*: People who snack on nuts may have less abdominal fat compared to those who munch on carb-based snacks. Nuts have monounsaturated fats—a heart healthier (and more satisfying) pick than their snack drawer counterparts (bye for now, pretzels!). Make sure you stick to the unsalted versions to stave off salt-induced bloating. Remember: A 1-ounce serving of nuts is about 170 calories (and can add up quickly), so use a small handful as your gauge.

   - **Try it:** Almonds, peanuts, walnuts, cashews are all great, but my favorite are shelled pistachios; they've got all the benefits, and the simple act of having to de-shell them helps to naturally slow you down (30 pistachios = about 100 calories).

6. **Limit the "sugar-free" stuff.** It's no secret that sugar substitutes—both natural and artificial—can lead to uncomfortable tummy troubles like gas and bloating. But some, like sugar-free gum and diet soda, work overtime: Since both carbonation and air bubbles you take in while chewing (or sipping from a straw) can contribute to gas production, you're better off steering clear of these items when you're looking to stop bloating in its tracks. Take note: Sugar alcohols can be sneaky bloat inducers found in packaged foods and baked goods, so check product labels for words ending in "-tol": sorbitol, xylitol, and erythritol.

Road Food 101

Let these be your go-to shortcuts for boosting satiety, cutting bloat, and generally feeling better when you travel: Be choosy about *where* you eat *which* foods. Remember how "self-care" requires *boundaries* and all of *that*? When you're traveling (especially internationally!) every meal can become a chance to take part in a shared experience and learn more about a new culture that can inspire your regular routine once you return home. Plus, prioritizing "must-try" restaurants and local specialties is *its own framework* from which to make all of your *other* food choices! For example: *You're in Paris! You want CREPES. You want NUTELLA CREPES! So by all means*: Make that choice, and allow that to provide you with a framework for your other choices throughout the day—do you *need* the sandwich right now after your Musée D'Orsay tour, or can you have a piece of fruit now, hit the Louvre, and save it for those Nutella crepes *later*? Intentionality and prioritization help you make the most nutritious choice or the most *special* food choice in any scenario—zero deprivation required.

Carry-on 3–2–1

Bring 3+ small snack items you (pretty much) always like to eat:

- Combo of portable protein: cheese sticks; hard-boiled eggs; unsweetened Greek yogurt, or a lower-sugar sweetened version—for example, Siggi's dairy (any), Chobani Greek (pumpkin spice); Oikos Triple Zero (any, but the plain is pretty sweet-tasting, so your best bet is to stick with that and add on from there). The Good Culture cottage cheese is another great pick as an alternative to yogurt.
- Fly-high fiber: veggies, unsweetened dried fruit, nuts, seeds, and trail mix, which also provide that mix, as do 100 percent whole grains and pulse snacks, like roasted chickpeas from Biena and The Good Bean, roasted edamame from Eda-Zen, lentil flour–based crackers from Saffron Road, and Rule Breaker brownies (which are made from black bean flour!).
- Stick-to-your ribs fat: peanut butter, almond butter, trail mix, cheese, whole-milk dairy products, eggs, and popcorn.

- Alternatively, something comfy-ish: popcorn, kettle-cooked potato chips, 3–5 minis of chocolate, CIBO Express box of sweetness, peanut M&M's.

Cheese Snacks

Sargento Balanced Breaks: I love these as both a snack and a teaching tool, because they're a great way to learn what a good, *actually balanced* snack looks like!

Jerky

ATTN: Travelers! Processed meat sticks (and slices) with health halos ("non-GMO!" "organic! "gluten-free!") are still Slim Jims! True, jerky *is* a real food and it *is* high protein, both of which are key indicators of something that could be beneficial for zapping FNSS. Ones that are made from lower-fat cuts of beef (like top round) or other animals (like turkey) can be A-OK for a snack—especially when combined with a piece of fruit for some extra fiber. That said, they're not always your best choice across the board: Jerky can be filled with sodium and saturated fat by nature of what it *is*—cured, aka *processed* meat (regularly eating too much of this is linked to increasing your risk of chronic disease in the long-term, but for the short-term, it's particularly linked to sadness when you realize you're flying into Parma, Italy, and are taken straight to the origin of *prosciutto di Parma*!!! Save it for the best source if you're heading there or somewhere similar *already*, right?

However, since airports seem to go nuts over jerky, and at other times, it may be your only option, let's make it work!

- Look for versions with as few ingredients as possible and aim to cap sodium and saturated fat at 230 mg and 3 g, respectively.
- Cap flavored types at 4 g or 1 teaspoon of sugar per serving.
- Grab a banana to balance that salt with some potassium, the mineral counterbalance, and make sure you're not going into a flight dehydrated or with your blood pressure up a teensy bit.

When you can opt out of that meat stick, some other great jerky alternatives that are super trendy right now: Fruit- and veggie-based versions, which you can find en route during travel (or order online) before you pack:

- Fruit jerky (Peeled Snacks—spicy mango is LIT)
- Laughing Giraffe Organics
- Trader Joe's, Whole Foods

Two 16-ounce beverages (seriously)

This should be in the form of one 16-ounce bottle of plain or sparkling water and one bottle (or cup) of something else unsweetened—like coffee if it's a morning flight; iced tea, unsweetened lemonade, or some sort of Bai/LaCroix/Spindrift/CORE/something tasty. I know, you're rolling your eyes at me—I can feel it from my middle seat all the way back here *IN the toilet*—but listen up: *altitude is dehydrating.* (And you know how you get when you're thirsty.)

#protip

Staying hydrated in-flight is the best way to offset the following feelings:

Hanger; hunger; fury; jet lag; crankiness; in-flight muscle cramps; travel-induced constipation; alcohol-induced ineptitude upon landing.

Bottom line: The longer you fly, the more water you need—and regardless of (a) how anxious you are, (b) how exhausted you are, and (c) how much you hate getting out of your middle seat to wait in the bathroom line, aka my satellite office: Think of your in-flight hydration game as literally just that—an actual skill to be honed, developed, and mastered.

One piece or one prepackaged snack bag of produce

Board the plane with one fresh item for you and a piece of produce for any/all family members. (Your produce pick is like your oxygen mask. I mean, how else are you supposed to help anyone else in case of a fruit-less emergency if you're not both hydrated and comfortably sated!? You really *cannot*.)

Good items for travel are apples and pears because they're less messy than, say, a mushy banana that explodes at the bottom of your carry-on, and less of a hassle than an orange when the juice spritzes into the eye of your seatmate...but I digress. Veggies work for this, too—I actually saw someone eating an onion like an apple in the customs line recently, and it was absolutely enlightening! (I don't think eating at customs is allowed...but that was one *badass bitch*!)

Social media often would have you believe that all of us have *oodles* of time to do things like cut up broccoli florets and put them into portable Tupperware before a flight. And really, if you do have time to do such things, I hope you'll come and teach me your ways! Until we meet: Never mind that Pinterest-perfect noise—the airport has plenty of goodies from which to choose these days.

MCDONALD'S 101

Call me crazy, but is there actually anything better in the world than McDonald's French fries?! Okay, I guess you're right. But drive-throughs like these can have a time and a place, and often that place is on a road trip with family, friends, or Bob from accounting (whom, since Tuscaloosa, you've deemed a pretty decent driver—well done, Bob!).

Classic Hamburger or Cheeseburger

Nutrition stats:

Hamburger: 250 calories, 3 g saturated fat, 480 mg sodium, 13 g protein, 2 g fiber

Cheeseburger: 300 calories, 5 g saturated fat, 680 mg sodium, 15 g protein, 2 g fiber

Here's the thing about burgers: They've gotten a bad rap over the years because of their super-sizing, double-patty-ing, and general ability to serve as a vehicle for melted cheese, bacon, or both. But at McDonald's, the "trick" is in the portion size, making a classic burger one of your better choices—hands down!

It delivers 13 g protein at only 250 calories per serving. Add flavor with pickles, onions, mustard, and a little bit of BBQ sauce or ketchup. If you're making a full meal out of it: Add a side salad to deliver some extra produce (and hearty, fiber-filled veggie serving!) to add bulk to your meal, helping you stay fuller, longer.

If you are in the market for a cheesier edition, the cheeseburger's not your worst choice. The cheese brings this bad boy to 300 calories and 5 g (versus 3 g) of saturated fat, and it will set you back by 680 mg sodium (about a quarter of your daily value); but if you're looking for a better-for-you version of the extra-large, greasy fast-food options: A McD's cheeseburger is one of your best bets.

Kids' Fries

Nutrition stats: 110 calories, 80 mg sodium, 1 g protein, 1 g fiber

It's great for…when you're desperate for fries but also want a burger.

Fries—much like burgers!—only deserve a bad rap for ginormous portion size (and their tendency to live under a pile of melted cheese), not just for nutritional quality. The kids' fries are a smart choice—they're relatively low in calories and are a low-sodium food (yes, really! The FDA defines a low-sodium food as 140 mg or less), so thanks to the serving size, the burger-and-fries meal you're in the mood for is ready and waiting.

Artisan Grilled Chicken Sandwich

Nutrition stats: 380 calories, 2 g saturated fat, 1,110 mg sodium, 11 g sugar, 37 g protein

It's great for…when you want a sandwich but you're surrounded by extra-large subs, paninis, and grease.

When you're in a bind (e.g., food court, road trip, airport, or simply have a hankering for a hearty, filling chicken sandwich), this one's pretty A-OK. That's because it'll keep you full for hours, thanks to a whopping 37 g of protein for just 380 calories—most extra-large sandwiches, subs, and paninis just start at 500 calories a pop. Since the chicken is marinated (and not deep-fried, greased, or cheese-laden), it's also lower in saturated fat, without sacrificing flavor. Keep in mind: If you're watching your salt, this may be a sandwich to skip: It's got 1,110 mg sodium (half of your daily value). But compared to its sub, roll, and flatbread counterparts: It's 100 percent a win. Balance out the salt with potassium-packed Cuties and at least 16 ounces of water.

Egg White Delight McMuffin/Egg McMuffin

Nutrition stats: Egg McMuffin: 300 calories, 6 g saturated fat, 730 mg sodium, 18 g protein, 2 g fiber

Egg-white Delight McMuffin: 260 calories, 4.5 g saturated fat, 750 mg sodium, 16 g protein, 2 g fiber

Now that McDonald's has breakfast all day, you can enjoy eggs at any time—and the McMuffin is a breakfast classic, no matter what time of day! Starting your day with a greater amount of protein (20 g is ideal, and these are both pretty close!) can help you stave off FNSS later on. When you're on the road, this is a better alternative than sugary fruit and yogurt parfait or premade, sweetened oatmeal. They're energy-boosting breakfasts that are lower in protein (just 6 g max!) and upward of 22 g sugar (5.5 teaspoons!). Pair this sammie with fruit, drink plenty of H_2O throughout the day to stay hydrated, and nix the processed meat from lunch and dinner (unless, of course, you're on that flight to Italy, in which case you can make an exception).

Jet Lag–Defying Snack Strategies

Base your time-traveling snacking on the following constants (conveniently, these are also located on the seat-back in front of you!):

- Time at point of origin
- Time at destination
- Flight duration

MORNING FLIGHT, 5–6 HOURS WITH TIME CHANGE BACKWARD (EST → PST)

This is easily the most difficult flight to, ahem, navigate from a nutritional standpoint, but there are a few important tricks, concepts, and ideas to put in place to ensure you make the most of this beautiful gift of time. (*WHEN ELSE DO WE EVER GET THREE EXTRA WHOLE HOURS?! This flight is a gift!!*) Think about using this flight, aka the time capsule, as a place that you can use to do *whatever* you want to do—sleep a little, work a little, and have a project, such as a movie, magazine, dream journal, knitting, or even a book (remember, you can ~~preorder~~ buy *and* read multiple copies of this one to reread it midair!!)—and it is so damn beautiful when it leaves early in the morning, because you've got a solid three hours up there before people at work start heckling you.

So consider your eating strategy your marathon fuel. What are you going to eat to boost energy, stay alert, and finish what you want to finish on this flight? If you're staying up: two-part breakfast or lunch; have a snack packed (in your seat pocket) for initial descent (if you need it).

TRANSCONTINENTAL FLIGHT (WITH A TIME CHANGE MOVING BACKWARD (EST → PST)

This is another power hour of magic, because if you're leaving during a peak work hour for you in the time zone you're leaving, you can get sh*t done without your inbox going nonstop, energy/time vampires invading your office, or the need to stop what you're doing to get something to eat. Have at least one meal before you board the plane, depending on the time of your travel, and stay on top of that hydration (of course!). Stick to your every three- or four-hour plan with your carry-on snacks, but, depending on how far you're going and what you're doing when you land, time a meal (or a sneal) two to three hours before touchdown (two hours if you've got time to check in before dinner with clients) and three hours before if you're going straight from the airport.

TRANSATLANTIC FLIGHT AT NIGHT WITH A TIME CHANGE MOVING FORWARD (UNITED STATES → EUROPE)

Get yourself a sneal two to three hours before the flight, either one you've packed or one you can find at a lounge (if you're fancy like that) or something you can pick up in the airport.

EVENING FLIGHT OF TEN OR MORE HOURS WITH ANY TIME CHANGE

For this one, take three-plus snacks and two components of a meal, such as the type of yogurt you like at breakfast; the type of bar you'd eat if you didn't have time for breakfast; a homemade PB&J in your carry-on; etc. that you have sitting in a cooler in the compartment above your head.

TRAVEL DELAYS: NOW WHAT?

For every hour you're delayed and hungry, consider going up in calories by the 100-calorie marker. For example, you're delayed an hour, and you were planning on having a little sneal when you got on the plane. Grab a piece of fruit, for about 100 calories, to tide you over. You're delayed two hours, opt for one of your carry-on snacks, for 200 calories.

HELP! I'M AWAY FROM HOME AND I FEEL LIKE I'M COMING DOWN WITH SOMETHING!

There's a lot of bogus claims out there about staying healthy while you travel. These are the top nutrition-related myths that come my way (and a few ideas about what to try instead).

1. **Drink fruit or veggie juices and smoothies when sick.** Skip juices and smoothies entirely—the blood sugar crash will only make you feel worse, and you're not reaping the same benefits as you would if you ate the food itself, which is higher in fiber, phytonutrients, and prebiotics, all linked to improved health and well-being. A better swap:

tea and—gasp—even coffee! (It's the #1 source of antioxidants in the American diet!) Other ways to give yourself a boost: Add extra veggies to salads, sandwiches, soups, sautés, and omelets or egg scrambles, and stick with water and seltzer for hydration. When you're feeling under the weather, veggie soup, stew, and broths (which can provide immune-boosting amino acids and minerals) can be soothing, while the heat helps open up congestion.

2. **Your body needs more antioxidants to help you stay healthy** while traveling. In food form, yes. But in pill or supplement form, absolutely not. Most antioxidants are water soluble, which means that whatever you're *not* using, you're excreting through urine. Other types of antioxidants, like vitamins A and E, are fat soluble, which means that they are stored in your body for prolonged periods. That means that it's (a) difficult to be deficient in them on the diets we typically eat today, and (b) supplementation of antioxidants can have a prooxidative effect (causing harm to cells instead of protecting them). Long-term studies have linked supplementation of these nutrients to certain types of lifestyle-related cancers, so definitely *avoid*! If you're *already* sick, adding extra vitamin C onto your daily dose won't help you heal any faster, but a zinc lozenge *may* help out on the back end: 15 mg twice a day has been linked to reducing duration of your cold, and at the very least, it can help scratchy throats feel better! Your body *does* have higher protein and fluid needs when you've got a fever. Lean protein from fish, eggs, nuts, seeds, beans, and lean cuts of beef and poultry are ideal. Make sure you're eating high-water fruits and veggies and drinking a *ton* of fluids—at least 10 cups per day from unsweetened sources.

3. **Echinacea will stop you from getting sick.** Replace this concept with a newer, better one: Consider a prophylactic probiotic all year round, which has been linked to reducing the duration of a cold and may help you stay healthier overall, decreasing your likelihood of getting sick. Eating foods rich in probiotic cultures (fermented foods, like sauerkraut and miso), and choosing Greek yogurt that has at least five strains of bacterial cultures added to it can also help your gut and immune system be healthier. Lastly, use common sense to take care of yourself all year round. Be sure to wash your hands, get enough sleep, and eat foods

high in prebiotic fiber (tons of colorful fruits and veggies), which can help boost immunity by starting where it matters most—your GI tract.

4. **I should have B vitamins to keep my energy up, right?** Yes, but only if you're *deficient* in B vitamins, which we haven't seen since the earth was cooling (or if you have Wernicke's encephalopathy, a condition that comes with either thiamin deficiency or alcohol poisoning—in which case I'm pretty sure you can't read the words in this book). Bottom line: It's likely not *you* with a deficiency in a B vitamin—so long as you eat your vegetables.

11

I've Been on a Diet for So Long, I'm Honestly Afraid of How I'll Look and Feel When I'm *Not* "Dieting"

After this chapter, you will...

- make peace with food (or at least begin the process).

"I can't go to dinner tonight because I'm on a diet." "I'm on (insert trendy diet name here), but I can sit with you and have water." "I'll have the side salad as my main, but *THE DRESSING MUST BE ON THE SIDE*! No croutons!" All of the many exhausting diet "rules" have proven unsuccessful and anxiety-inducing for the long haul. Restriction is not the recipe for success. And if you really did find at one point in your life that you *loved* plain, raw kale leaves, you might still wind up deficient in *nutrients* (without a little dressing on your kale, how are you going to absorb all of those antioxidants?). The *best* diets from around the globe (Mediterranean, Nordic, Middle Eastern, Central/ South American, and other cultures) are the ones that encourage a *lifestyle* that celebrates health through food: growing, picking, prepping, eating, and enjoying food in ways that honor your physical body, your spirit, and your mental health. Eating "right" or "well" means sharing experiences through food that promote happiness and fulfillment—whatever that means for *you*.

I totally get it. This seems a little hard to you at first! But I promise, that's the way it's supposed to feel when you're getting ready to make real, lasting change that will work for you for the rest of your life!

We've spent ten whole "counseling sessions" together on these pages, and now here we are at the root of it—you are concerned about what it really means to let go of restrictions and associated phrases like *cutting back* and *eliminating* and *-free!*; plus *fasting, juicing, no carbs! no fat! keto! paleo!* and *vegan!* are hereby a thing of the past!

"I Don't Know If I Can Do This!" (and Other Lies We Tell Ourselves)

Truth time: There is a sense of loneliness and isolation when it comes to making substantial changes to the way you think about and take real agency in your personal health—especially because today's diet-driven culture has a sense of "we're in this together!" camaraderie that develops among "dieters" (especially come Q1 of a new year!). So let me be clear: *I know this isn't easy!* And I also completely understand why you're afraid—*doing less* is often not the path of least resistance that it may seem!

But I also know this: Above all else, when it comes to your mental and physical health, weight, and emotional well-being, diets are a program for self-doubt, feelings of abandonment, and shame. Diets have made you feel helpless, inert, and out of control—and there's nothing more lonely or isolating than believing that you "can't" or you "should" or that to take action and see positive change, you need to be someone different from who you are *right now*!

To make changes for the rest of your life, you have to start small, keep it simple, and do what's right for you—*you are your number one priority*! And to really put these words into action, you need a plan that is manageable within the framework of who you are, what you do, and where you spend your time—all day, every day. Making positive changes to your health means that the process has to feel just as good as the end goal.

"I Am Afraid of Failing at This"

Making better food choices and being on a diet (in any traditional sense of the way we use that word) are *different things*. A growing body of research (beginning in the early 2000s) has come out showing that an overweight BMI is not necessarily an indicator of health status—especially when your blood sugar, cholesterol, and blood pressure are normal. This is a great thing in many ways, and the ongoing research and development of body positivity and weight acceptance is invaluable to changing the narrative about what "health" actually means. Overall, the message is generally beneficial—*every single one of us* could benefit from feeling mentally and physically good about ourselves no matter how much we weigh and no matter what size we wear.

However.

The collateral damage of the "anti–body shaming" and "anti–diet culture" movement is often anyone and everyone who wants to make better food choices, take ownership of their health, and *yes*—lose weight. This rising stigma is a newer, subtler, rebranded form of shame, and an offshoot of traditional diet culture, all dressed up in a "mind, body, spirit!" costume. To me, this doesn't feel like significant progress. Working to improve *actual, powerful, and long-lasting well-being,* from both a mental *and* physical health perspective, does not *only* mean "having a better body image" but it also means consistently developing and honing the confidence to take health-promoting action that *works for you as an individual,* in the context of your everyday life—without the scrutiny, judgment, and blame of those who choose to do it differently.

Shame of *any kind* breeds feelings of isolation and loneliness— feelings that play a tremendous role in our public health conversation today (some studies have linked social isolation to mortality in ways that are on par with smoking statistics). If better health could be achieved by restricting, eliminating, calorie counting, detoxing, cleansing, supplementing, portion controlling, and "everything in moderation"-ing, *wouldn't they be working by now? Wouldn't we be happier, healthier, better versions of ourselves? And wouldn't we have sustained that for longer than a year (max)?! I rest my case!* They would! Which means, they've *already failed you.* (*Glad we got that out of the way.*)

Without a set meal plan or ascribed value system for judging food, it's easy to feel *super vulnerable.* You're driving—and that feels like a lot of responsible choices that need to get made in a row! So to offset all of that fear, let's break this down to the most basic recap of *all of the strategies* we've learned so far so that you can feel comfortable taking on new challenges, or scaling back a few steps when you need to:

- **Stop giving food the upper hand in your relationship.** Forget about "good" or "bad" foods. Remember that your state of health changes by making better, more nutritious food choices *most of the time*—it's not going to fly out the window based on one meal, one day, one week! There isn't such a thing as "messing this up," because overdoing it sometimes is a part of life, and living life = your new "meal plan." Look at you! You're *killing it*!

- **Use personal policies to combat boundary bullies.** Protect your own personal brand of self-care. Boundary bullies are only as successful as you allow them to be. Remember that you are in charge of establishing who and what deserves your time and attention, even when obligation rears its ugly head. Protect your priorities as they relate to taking care of yourself by planning ahead and setting a standard for the things you won't do in order to check off items on the list of things you want more, or things that make you, personally, feel better.

- **Resist the urge to throw a pity party.** Spoiler alert: You *will* overeat sometimes. You will eat sugar when you weren't planning to eat dessert. You will sometimes skip breakfast and wind up hoarding donuts in your desk drawer. SO. WHAT? *No one is immune to the realities of everyday life.* You will not derail your own state of health as a result of a meal or a day of eating all of the things, and staying in the exact same place. Therefore, you are *not* going to throw a pity party and bring in all of your demons to beat you up over being a human being. Doing *that* sets us up for failure because it brings back all of the shame, all of the isolation, and makes us feel like we are all alone in the world—all because we did something that every human does sometimes! It's the guilty mind-set that *will* make you gain weight. Being healthier, happier, and losing (and maintaining) weight is not a 100 percent immovable set point or place in time that you have to "get to" in order to be happier and healthier.

- **Use the three T's to help you navigate any food-focused "barrier" that comes your way.** Making better choices becomes a habit over time.

The more you do it, the more comfortable you will be, and the more instinctual it will become to make choices that leave you feeling your best.

- **Type:** All of your meals are made from the satiety trifecta: protein, fiber, and healthy fats.
- **Timing:** You eat breakfast every day, and you eat consistently after that: every three to four hours.
- **Tools:** Keep yourself full and satisfied by preparing ahead of time to have the supplies you need on hand, whether you're on your regular routine or on the road. The more often you prepare ahead, the more it will become second nature! When in doubt: More vegetables, more movement.

■ **Stick to your vision, but be flexible within the plan.** Your vision is better health. Your boundaries help you prioritize accordingly in ways that actually allow you to act on it. Use your Ulysses contract: When you might *not* make it to a workout class today, what will you do instead? If you're going out and planning to drink *all of the champagne, because YOLO*, what do you need to eat that day and at dinner that night in order to not *want* to consume the entire contents of your fridge? If you have "no time for breakfast," well…you sure as heck better be implementing a two-part breakfast solution. Your health-focused priorities are similar to the foods you eat: What matters is what you do most of the time. Being flexible with yourself and making choices that lift you up is a habit you deserve to form.

■ **Remember that you are only responsible for your choices.** When something is seemingly irresistible, remind yourself that you have a *choice* (and one of the options is eating that irresistible thing and LOVING it). Check in with yourself to see if you're feeling powerless because of any of these triggers:

- You're dehydrated.
- You have an empty stomach/skipped a meal/skipped breakfast/ didn't eat enough for breakfast.
- You didn't sleep enough/aren't sleeping enough in general.
- You've made a change in your regular exercise routine that is throwing off your appetite.

And if it *is* one of those: That's okay! The first two you can tackle in the moment by (a) drinking something unsweetened, and (b) eating a meal or a snack or a sneal. But do both of those first, and then make the decision. Reminder: *Going for it* is a decision that you want to make for yourself, so whenever you can, optimize your set of circumstances and don't try to reason with a dehydrated, low-blood-sugar version of yourself.

- **Eat more produce.** When in doubt, add vegetables. You can literally ignore everything else in this book if it all feels like *too much for you* at a given moment; just choose more fruit and more vegetables every time you eat, and you're *already on the right track* to better health. The *more* you eat veggies, the *greater* the portion of veggies on your plate... displacing the amount of other food that is higher in calories and may not be as nutritious—but you're still *actually chewing*, and getting actual, real fiber that helps you fill up. And on the fruit side of the spectrum: Forget about all of the things you've learned before you read this book that fruit is "high in sugar!" or that it has to be "cold pressed" and "juiced!" If you need a strategy for doing this *right away*, you can make all of your snacks have at least one piece of fruit (or 1 cup of fruit), and make half of your plate vegetables at breakfast, lunch, and dinner. Voila! You're crushing it.

- **Eat more REAL dessert.** Added sugar is everywhere, so staying aware of where these sneaky sugar sources are coming from and how they're making their way into everything you formerly ate is going to help you make the conscious choice to eat dessert every single day. Look for treats in their delicious, wonderful, transparent glory: Frozen treats, candy, and baked goods that are single-serve, with easy-to-read, simple ingredients.

- **Eat more fish and pulses.** Ninety percent of us don't eat enough fish— which is a problem, because a lot of seafood is lean protein that's good for your brain and your heart. And if you are of childbearing age/ have children/ever think you might consider having children/can keep a houseplant alive, your offspring need the omega-3s found in seafood. For this, 8 to 12 ounces per week is your goal, and you can make it easier on yourself by choosing canned or frozen options or buying fresh from a fishmonger you trust. Another underconsumed food to prioritize for better health and better satiety? Pulses—beans, chickpeas, lentils, and peas—which give you fiber and protein and make any meal more affordable because they're plant based, not animal based.

- **When in doubt, *do less*.** An average Monday night meal does not need to be some three-course dining experience, nor does it have to be vegan, gluten-free, and dairy-free (but you *know that* by now!). Have bases on hand that you've already made in bulk, and use that to make customizable dinners that make *everyone* ~~less whiny~~ happier. Reminder: The key word is *bar*. Pasta bar, potato bar, sandwich bar, taco bar—anything can be a bar if you provide enough toppings! In other words, use shortcuts whenever and wherever you can in ways that do all of the things we've covered in this book. A little resourcefulness goes a long way, and food technology can help you get it done when you need just that (precut veggies, single-serve items, frozen cauliflower rice = food technology). And this is the technology age, people! So do less, and take advantage of what's out there!

"I Don't Know If I Can Handle the Emotional Turmoil of Losing and Gaining Weight Again"

Start by being honest with yourself. It's key for long-term weight loss and health success that *most* of your choices start *from the right place*. Every client I have ever met with for the purpose of weight loss was, at some point, not doing the best they could in staying on top of *one or more* of these strategies.

Traditional weight loss and diet culture promises that restriction in the present will lead to happiness in the *future*. The opposing body-positivity-gone-awry culture makes accepting your current physicality the *only* route to health and happiness. IMO, neither of these promote holistic health—be it mental or physical.

After honesty comes *reframing*: Okay, so let's say (*purely hypothetical situation here!*) that you are a regular exerciser who considers yourself a regular "gym-goer," runner, exerciser who is trying to do a *decent* job at your (rather demanding!) job in a constantly changing industry;

responsible for showing up to your *second job* (less demanding, but arguably just as time-consuming!) and responsible for maintaining (at least 50 percent!) of the relationship you have with every *other human being in your life*; attempting to be a caregiver for parents, grandparents, siblings, children, pets, houseplants—you name it, you're probably responsible for their well-being, amirite? And on top of all of *that*: You thought you were going to use the time you thought you'd finally have to watch *Stranger Things* on Netflix, and instead, you go ahead and take on *another* work project; adopt *another* puppy; decide to have *children*; decide *not to have children*—you name it. You made a life choice or you underwent a life-changing event and that sh*t is HUGE.

And frankly, you just *do not have time* for exercise in the way you once did a few months ago, 100 percent of the time, every single day, or every single week! But does that mean you give up or stop *moving* in a way that feels like the best you can do for where you're at *right now*? No way, Jose. You *reframe*. You may not be running as much as you did last year, but does it mean you're doing the most *moving* you can possibly do for where you, personally, are at right now? Yes! Maybe under these circumstances, you're walking to and from work and the grocery store! And it turns out that you actually relish this time because it allows you to listen to lots of books *while you walk* and turn your brain off for just a sec! See how that works? You now have the tools you need to *reframe* your current way of thinking as it relates to your health and your time. There are always going to be difficult circumstances that come up in your life that challenge the notion that your own personal health is your top priority, but how you navigate those challenges is how you stay in a healthier, happier place for *life*.

This book encourages you to think about health as it relates not only to how you feel in the present and how you'd like to feel in some very distant future, but also how you personally *want to feel* in an hour, two hours, two days, two weeks. So if any of the changes we've talked about aren't making you feel generally *good* about the choices you're making at any given moment, it's time to either *do less* or *reframe* based on where you're at, and consider what piece of the process isn't working for you.

Eating real food and sharing meals and experiences among loved ones should be joyful, fulfilling, and enriching. (And that, my friends, is the definition of health and happiness.) Now you know that practice builds confidence, and confidence builds habits—you've built a lot of this foundation already, and you have the tools to make these habits solid for the rest of your life in a way that will result in sustained weight loss (and ultimately, weight maintenance). Never forget that no one knows what's best for you better than you do.

So, promise me this: No more ordering dressing on the side, asking for burgers without the bun, or missing out on experiences because you're "on a diet," okay?

It's those handcuffs from which (I hope!) this book has *set you free*.

Acknowledgments

Hey, *you*. Yes, *YOU*, reader of this book: I just want to say, *thanks for being here!*

Thank you for showing up, staying the course, and heeding the advice on these pages in whatever way works best for you, in the context of your incredibly dynamic, nuanced, and wholly unique everyday *life*! Without *you*, this book would not exist, and for that I am both overwhelmingly grateful and completely humbled. So, one more time, *for the cheap seats in the back*: I appreciate you, I believe in *you*, and I can't thank you enough for believing in *me*.

There are a slew of authors whom I greatly admire who have extolled the benefits of having "*a* mentor"; I am fortunate enough to say that I have *many*, all of whom have inspired me with their wisdom, compassion, and grace.

First and foremost, my brilliant, empathetic, passionate, hilarious, inspiring, talented (*I could keep going with the adjectives, but she would probably edit me by a hundred words*) editor at Grand Central, Leah Miller—I am forever grateful to you and your brain, and for becoming a navigator and translator for *my* (highly jumbled!) brain. You are a unicorn for *so* many reasons *thatihavenospacelefttowrite*, and I am so lucky to know you.

A tremendous thanks, too, to the entire Grand Central team for your incredible work on turning these words into an *actual book*! (*Amazing, right?!*)

To this end, I must give all of that credit where it's due: my boys, Dado Derviskadic and Steve Troha, my agents at Folio Literary Management—my true champions since day one, which is, by the way, *quite* some time ago now. (*Funny, we haven't aged a day...!*) Thanks for tracking me down, for believing in me, and for knowing *exactly where, how, and with whom* this vision would come to life. It's time for a *seriously overdue* cocktail.

To my colleagues and friends at *Good Housekeeping* who have, without fail, stood in my corner throughout this process and who cultivate an environment in which both scientific analysis and expansive, creative thinking *thrive*. Writing and editing this book would not have happened without all of you, especially my second family (aka, the GH Institute). I am better every day because of *you*.

For all of you who have generously planted the seeds from which this work has blossomed, THANK YOU—especially *you*: Lisa Sasson, Sara Wilson (+ all the RDs—past and present—with whom I've had the privilege of working and learning from at Mount Sinai), Willow Jarosh, Lauren Antonucci, Barbara Linhardt, Jo Bartell, Jen White, and so many more who inspire me daily (near and far). And since we're on the topic of RDs...an extra-ginormous, all-caps THANK YOU to the amazing Danielle Zolotnitsky, my former-intern-turned-researcher for this book (and beyond!). Danielle is like a nutrition information oracle, and one of the greatest researchers, most talented practitioners, and an all-around excellent person to hang out with/get to know. (If you live in the greater Philadelphia area: Go find her, people!) This could not have happened without you—*thank you* for your relentlessness. I'm in your corner, always!

For my friends: *I hope you're still there? I finished my book! Let's hang out...?!* All I can say is I love you and I can't believe you put up with me, especially my HLP, Maegan (+ David!!!) Morris (who *really* was the primary instigator of this whole "writing a book" thing): You are my person and my sister. Maggie Tsai, Eimear Lynch, and Erin Nemser, my emotional cornerstones, and the boys—Nick, Pete, Mike, Greg: Milk thistle is *still not a thing* (just in case you thought I'd forget...well, I *didn't*.)

To my boyfriend, Michael: Remember when you told me you weren't "looking for anything serious"? I sure do! Thanks for (a) appreciating my slightly deranged sense of humor and (b) taking care of our four-legged *kids* in our *shared apartment* as I sit here and type *these* acknowledgments! Love you!

At the top of the list, A-number-one: This book is, above all else, for my family. I wrote *Dressing on the Side* during one of the scariest, loneliest, most difficult periods of my life—one that remains unpredictable in nature as we go to press.

With that in mind, since we never *really know* how many more chances we'll get to say "thank you" and "I love you" to the people we cherish and appreciate the most, let me use this public forum to say just *that* to my family, near and far, extended (Erdheims!) and biological (I love you, Aunt Lolly!!).

Above all else, especially, the Griswolds (Nan, Stace, Toria, and Deanst): I LOVE YOU. THANK YOU. I am eternally grateful for sharing DNA, tears, laughter, generalized anxiety, imagination, creativity, humor, sour-gummy candy, and a deep-seated, profound passion for all things *Barry Manilow* with *you*! (I just can't smile without you, fam!)

Finally, for *you*, Dad: You are the single bravest person this world has ever known. You really *are* Superman; you really *are* the funniest, smartest, most inspiring public servant, thinker, writer, teacher, father, friend, leader, and my best "buddy"; you are *the human definition* of the phrase *one of a kind*. You have instilled in me an unwavering, unrelenting *inability* to turn my back on a challenge, and this book is a totem of *that* fact. So, thank you for reading it. Thank you for teaching me that true courageousness means MAPTO—going for the things you want, even when you didn't think you could do it, and even when you're terrified to try. I hope this book makes you proud; I'm sorry about all of the "foul language"; I love you more than anything—you're my hero, D.

Bibliography

"Added Sugars." American Heart Association. February 1, 2017. Accessed June 2018. https://www.heart.org/HEARTORG/HealthyLiving/Healthy Eating/Nutrition/Added-Sugars_UCM_305858_Article.jsp.

"Advisory: Replacing Saturated Fat with Healthier Fat Could Lower Cardiovascular Risks." News on Heart.org. June 22, 2017. https://news .heart.org/advisory-replacing-saturated-fat-with-healthier-fat-could -lower-cardiovascular-risks/.

An, R., and Y. Shi. "Consumption of Coffee and Tea with Add-ins in Relation to Daily Energy, Sugar, and Fat Intake in US Adults, 2001–2012." *Public Health* 146 (2017): 1–3. doi:10.1016/j.puhe.2016.12.032.

Angelopoulos, Theodore J., et al. "Fructose Containing Sugars at Normal Levels of Consumption Do Not Effect Adversely Components of the Metabolic Syndrome and Risk Factors for Cardiovascular Disease." *Nutrients* 8, no. 4 (2016): 179. *PMC*. Web. September 26, 2018.

"Artificial Sweeteners and Cancer." National Cancer Institute. May 2016. https://www.cancer.gov/about-cancer/causes-prevention/risk/diet/ artificial-sweeteners-fact-sheet.

Aune, Dagfinn, Edward Giovannucci, Boffetta Paolo, et al. "Fruit and Vegetable Intake and the Risk of Cardiovascular Disease, Total Cancer and All-Cause Mortality—a Systematic Review and Dose-Response Meta-analysis of Prospective Studies." *International Journal of Epidemiology* 46, no. 3 (2017): 1029–1056. doi:10.1093/ije/dyw319.

Aune, Dagfinn, NaNa Keum, Edward Giovannucci, et al. "Whole-Grain Consumption and Risk of Cardiovascular Disease, Cancer, and All Cause and Cause Specific Mortality: Systematic Review and Dose-Response Meta-analysis of Prospective Studies." *BMJ* 353, no. 2716 (2016). doi:10.1136/bmj.i2716.

Aune, Dagfinn, Deborah A. Navarro Rosenblatt, Doris S. M. Chan, et al. "Dairy Products, Calcium, and Prostate Cancer Risk: A Systematic Review and Meta-analysis of Cohort Studies." *American Journal of Clinical Nutrition* 101, no. 1 (2014): 87–117. doi:10.3945/ajcn.113.067157.

Balliett, Mary, and Jeanmarie R. Burke. "Changes in Anthropometric Measurements, Body Composition, Blood Pressure, Lipid Profile, and Testosterone in Patients Participating in a Low-energy Dietary Intervention." *Journal of Chiropractic Medicine* 12, no. 1 (2013): 3–14. doi:10.1016/j.jcm.2012.11.003.

Beheshti, Zahra, Yiong Huak Chan, Hamid Sharif Nia, et al. "Influence of Apple Cider Vinegar on Blood Lipids." *Life Science Journal* 9, no. 4 (2013): 2431–2440.

Bello, Alfonso E., and Steffen Oesser. "Collagen Hydrolysate for the Treatment of Osteoarthritis and Other Joint Disorders: A Review of the Literature." *Current Medical Research and Opinion* 22, no. 11 (2006): 2221–2232. doi:10.1185/030079906x148373.

Berryman, C. E., S. G. West, J. A. Fleming, P. L. Bordi, and P. M. Kris-Etherton. "Effects of Daily Almond Consumption on Cardiometabolic Risk and Abdominal Adiposity in Healthy Adults with Elevated LDL-Cholesterol: A Randomized Controlled Trial." *Journal of the American Heart Association* 4, no. 1 (2015). doi:10.1161/jaha.114.000993.

Bhupathiraju, S. N., D. K. Tobias, V. S. Malik, et al. "Glycemic Index, Glycemic Load, and Risk of Type 2 Diabetes: Results from 3 Large US Cohorts and an Updated Meta-analysis." *American Journal of Clinical Nutrition* 100, no. 1 (2014): 218–232. doi:10.3945/ajcn.113.079533.

Bradbury, Kathryn E., Paul N. Appleby, and Timothy J. Key. "Fruit, Vegetable, and Fiber Intake in Relation to Cancer Risk: Findings from the European Investigation into Cancer and Nutrition (EPIC)." *American Journal of Clinical Nutrition* 100, suppl 1 (July 2014): 394S–398S. doi.org/10.3945/ajcn.113.071357.

Brodesser-Akner, Taffy. "Losing It in the Anti-Dieting Age." *New York Times*. August 2, 2017. https://www.nytimes.com/2017/08/02/magazine/weight-watchers-oprah-losing-it-in-the-anti-dieting-age.html.

Cantu-Jungles, T. M., L. A. McCormack, J. E. Slaven, M. Slebodnik, and H. A. Eicher-Miller. "A Meta-Analysis to Determine the Impact of Restaurant Menu Labeling on Calories and Nutrients (Ordered or Consumed) in U.S. Adults." *Nutrients* 9, no. 10 (2017): 1088. doi:10.3390/nu9101088.

Cardoso, D. A., A. S. Moreira, G. M. de Oliveria, and G. Rosa. "A Coconut Extra Virgin Oil-Rich Diet Increases HDL Cholesterol and Decreases Waist Circumference and Body Mass in Coronary Artery Disease Patients." *Nutrición Hospitalaria* 5, no. 32 (November 1, 2015): 2144–2152. doi:10.3305/nh.2015.32.5.9642.

Center for Food Safety and Applied Nutrition. "Dietary Supplements." US Food and Drug Administration Home Page. June 25, 2015. Accessed June 2018. https://www.fda.gov/Food/DietarySupplements/.

Center for Food Safety and Applied Nutrition. "Food Additives & Ingredients—FDA Statement on European Aspartame Study." US Food and Drug Administration Home Page. April 20, 2007. Accessed May 2018. https://www.fda.gov/food/ingredientspackaginglabeling/foodaddit ivesingredients/ucm208580.htm.

Center for Food Safety and Applied Nutrition. "Food Additives & Ingredients—Final Determination Regarding Partially Hydrogenated Oils (Removing Trans Fat)." US Food and Drug Administration Home Page. May 5, 2018. Accessed June 2018. https://www.fda.gov/food/ingre dientspackaginglabeling/foodadditivesingredients/ucm449162.htm.

Center for Food Safety and Applied Nutrition. "Labeling & Nutrition—Changes to the Nutrition Facts Label." US Food and Drug Administration Home Page. Accessed May 2018. https://www.fda.gov/Food/GuidanceRegulation/GuidanceDocumentsRegulatoryInformation/LabelingNutrition/ucm385663.htm?utm_source=msn.

Center for Food Safety and Applied Nutrition. "Labeling & Nutrition—Guidance for Industry: Nutrition Labeling Manual—A Guide for Developing and Using Data Bases." US Food and Drug Administration Home Page. 1998. https://www.fda.gov/Food/GuidanceRegulation/GuidanceDocumentsRegulatoryInformation/LabelingNutrition/ucm063113.htm.

Center for Food Safety and Applied Nutrition. "Labeling & Nutrition—Industry Resources on the Changes to the Nutrition Facts Label." US Food and Drug Administration Home Page. June 14, 2018. https://www.fda.gov/Food/GuidanceRegulation/GuidanceDocumentsRegulatoryInformation/LabelingNutrition/ucm513734.htm.

Chung, M., J. Ma, K. Patel, S. Berger, J. Lau, and A. H. Lichtenstein. "Fructose, High-Fructose Corn Syrup, Sucrose, and Nonalcoholic Fatty Liver Disease or Indexes of Liver Health: A Systematic Review and

Meta-analysis." *American Journal of Clinical Nutrition* 100, no. 3 (2014): 833–849. doi:10.3945/ajcn.114.086314.

Cline, J. C. "Nutritional Aspects of Detoxification in Clinical Practice." *Alternative Therapies in Health and Medicine* 21, no. 3 (2015): 54–62. PubMed PMID: 26026145.

Coleman, Andrew M. *Dictionary of Psychology.* Oxford, England: Oxford University Press, 2003: Oxford University Press, 2015.

Del Gobbo, L. C., M. C. Falk., R. Feldman, K. Lewis, and D. Mozaffarian. "Effects of Tree Nuts on Blood Lipids, Apolipoproteins, and Blood Pressure: Systematic Review, Meta-analysis, and Dose-response of 61 Controlled Intervention Trials." *American Journal of Clinical Nutrition* 102, no. 6 (2015): 1347–1356. doi:10.3945/ajcn.115.110965.

Del Gobbo, L. C., F. Imamura, S. Aslibekyan, et al. "ω-3 Polyunsaturated Fatty Acid Biomarkers and Coronary Heart Disease: Pooling Project of 19 Cohort Studies." *JAMA Internal Medicine* 176, no. 8 (2016). doi:10.1001/jamainternmed.2016.2925.

De Souza, R. J., A. Mente, A. Maroleanu, et al. "Intake of Saturated and Trans Unsaturated Fatty Acids and Risk of All Cause Mortality, Cardiovascular Disease, and Type 2 Diabetes: Systematic Review and Meta-analysis of Observational Studies." *BMJ* 351, no. h3978 (2015). doi:10.1136/bmj.h3978.

"Dietary Guidelines for Americans 2015–2020 8th Edition." Chapter 4—2008 Physical Activity Guidelines. 2018. https://health.gov/dietary guidelines/2015/guidelines/.

"Division for Heart Disease and Stroke Prevention." Centers for Disease Control and Prevention. August 23, 2017. Accessed June 2018. https://www.cdc.gov/dhdsp/data_statistics/fact_sheets/fs_heart_disease.htm.

Donini, Lorenzo M., Lluis Serra-Majem, Mònica Bulló, Ángel Gil, and Jordi Salas-Salvadó. "The Mediterranean Diet: Culture, Health and Science." *British Journal of Nutrition* 113, no. S2 (2015). doi:10.1017/s0007114515001087.

Drewnowski, Adam, and Colin D. Rehm. "Consumption of Added Sugars Among US Children and Adults by Food Purchase Location and Food Source." *American Journal of Clinical Nutrition* 100, no. 3 (2014): 901–907. doi:10.3945/ajcn.114.089458.

Druesne-Pecollo, Nathalie, Paule Latino-Martel, et al. "Beta-carotene Supplementation and Cancer Risk: A Systematic Review and Metaanalysis of Randomized Controlled Trials." *International Journal of Cancer* 127, no. 1 (2009): 172–184. doi:10.1002/ijc.25008.

EatrightPRO, Academy of Nutrition and Dietetics. "What Is a Registered Dietitian Nutritionist." https://www.eatrightpro.org/about-us/what-is-an-rdn-and-dtr/what-is-a-registered-dietitian-nutritionist.

Fantino, Marc, Agnès Fantino, Marie Matray, and Frédéric Mistretta. "Beverages Containing Low Energy Sweeteners Do Not Differ from Water in Their Effects on Appetite, Energy Intake and Food Choices in Healthy, Non-obese French Adults." *Appetite* 125 (2018): 557–565. doi:10.1016/j.appet.2018.03.007.

Federal Trade Commission. "The FTC's Endorsement Guides: What People Are Asking." Federal Trade Commission. June 25, 2018. Accessed May 2018. https://www.ftc.gov/tips-advice/business-center/guidance/ftcs-endorsement-guides-what-people-are-asking.

"Food Allergy Research & Education® (FARE)." Food Allergy Research & Education. 2018. Accessed June 1, 2018. https://www.foodallergy.org/.

"Food Retail Implications for U.S. Grocery Shopper Trends." US Grocery Shopper Trends 2017. July 18, 2017. Food Retail Implications for U.S. Grocery Shopper Trends.

Foodsafety.gov. "Charts: Food Safety at a Glance." FoodSafety.gov. August 23, 2009. Accessed June 1, 2018. https://www.foodsafety.gov/keep/charts/index.html.

Forouhi, N. G., R. M. Krauss, G. Taubes, and W. Willett. "Dietary Fat and Cardiometabolic Health: Evidence, Controversies, and Consensus for Guidance." *BMJ* 361, no. k2139 (2018). doi:10.1136/bmj.k2139.

Galbete. C., J. Kröger, F. Jannasch, et al. "Nordic Diet, Mediterranean Diet, and the Risk of Chronic Diseases: the EPIC-Potsdam Study." *BMC Medicine* 16, no. 99 (2018). doi:10.1186/s12916-018-1082-y.

Gardner, Christopher D., John F. Trepanowski, Liana C. Del Gobbo, et al. "Effect of Low-Fat vs Low-Carbohydrate Diet on 12-Month Weight Loss in Overweight Adults and the Association with Genotype Pattern or Insulin Secretion." *JAMA* 319, no. 7 (2018): 667. doi:10.1001/jama.2018.0245.

Genetically Engineered Crops: Experiences and Prospects. Washington, DC: National Academies of Sciences, Engineering, and Medicine, 2016.

Ghasemian, Mona, Sina Owlia, and Mohammad Bagher Owlia. "Review of Anti-Inflammatory Herbal Medicines." *Advances in Pharmacological Sciences* 2016 (2016): 1–11. doi:10.1155/2016/9130979.

Gluten-Free Products Market Analysis by Product (Bakery, Dairy Alternatives, Desserts & Ice-Creams, Prepared Foods, Pasta & Rice), by Distribution (Grocery Stores, Mass Merchandiser, Club Stores), and Segment Forecasts, 2018–2025. Report no. GVR-1-68038-834-3. San Francisco: Grandview Research, 2017.

Griffiths, Keith, Bharat Aggarwal, Ram Singh, Harpal Buttar, Douglas Wilson, and Fabien De Meester. "Food Antioxidants and Their Anti-Inflammatory Properties: A Potential Role in Cardiovascular Diseases and Cancer Prevention." *Diseases* 4, no. 4 (2016): 28. doi:10.3390/diseases4030028.

Gupta, Divya. "Sleep and Alternative Medicine: I." Sleep Disorders Medicine, 2017, 1209–1220. doi:10.1007/978-1-4939-6578-6_56.

Hlebowicz, Joanna. "Effect of Apple Cider Vinegar on Delayed Gastric Emptying in People with Type 1 Diabetes Mellitus." http://isrctn.org/, 2013. doi:10.1186/isrctn33841495.

Holt-Lunstad, Julianne, Timothy B. Smith, Mark Baker, Tyler Harris, and David Stephenson. "Loneliness and Social Isolation as Risk Factors for Mortality." *Perspectives on Psychological Science* 10, no. 2 (2015): 227–237. doi:10.1177/1745691614568352.

Humphrey, Lauren, Dawn Clifford, and Michelle Neyman Morris. "Health at Every Size College Course Reduces Dieting Behaviors and Improves Intuitive Eating, Body Esteem, and Anti-Fat Attitudes." *Journal of Nutrition Education and Behavior* 47, no. 4 (2015). doi:10.1016/j.jneb.2015.01.008.

Khan, Tauseef A., and John L. Sievenpiper. "Controversies about Sugars: Results from Systematic Reviews and Meta-analyses on Obesity, Cardiometabolic Disease and Diabetes." *European Journal of Nutrition* 55, no. S2 (2016): 25–43. doi:10.1007/s00394-016-1345-3.

Kim, Shana J., Russell J. de Souza, Vivian L. Choo, et al. "Effects of Dietary Pulse Consumption on Body Weight: A Systematic Review and Meta-analysis of Randomized Controlled Trials." *American Journal of Clini-*

cal Nutrition 103, no. 5 (2016): 1213–1223, https://doi.org/10.3945/ajcn.115.124677.

Kind. "FDA Reverses Stance, Affirms KIND Can Use 'Healthy' on Its Labels | KIND Snacks." May 10, 2016. https://www.kindsnacks.com/media-center/press-releases/fda-reverses-stance.

Lee, Allen, and Chung Owyang. "Sugars, Sweet Taste Receptors, and Brain Responses." *Nutrients* 9, no. 7 (2017): 653. doi:10.3390/nu 9070653.

Liberman, Zoe, Amanda L. Woodward, Kathleen R. Sullivan, and Katherine D. Kinzler. "Early Emerging System for Reasoning about the Social Nature of Food." *Proceedings of the National Academy of Sciences* 113, no. 34 (2016): 9480–9485. doi:10.1073/pnas.1605456113.

Maalouf, J., M. E. Cogswell, J. P. Gunn, et al. "Monitoring the Sodium Content of Restaurant Foods: Public Health Challenges and Opportunities." *American Journal of Public Health* 103, no. 9 (2013): e21–e30. doi:10.2105/AJPH.2013.301442.

Manson, J. E., and S. S. Bassuk. "Vitamin and Mineral Supplements: What Clinicians Need to Know." *JAMA* 319, no. 9 (2018): 859–860. doi:10.1001/jama.2017.21012.

Marshall, Simon J., and Stuart J. H. Biddle. "The Transtheoretical Model of Behavior Change: A Meta-analysis of Applications to Physical Activity and Exercise." *Annals of Behavioral Medicine* 23, no. 4 (2001): 229–46. doi:10.1207/s15324796abm2304_2.

Mayhew, A., R. de Souza, D. Meyre, S. Anand, and A. Mente. "A Systematic Review and Meta-analysis of Nut Consumption and Incident Risk of CVD and All-Cause Mortality." *British Journal of Nutrition* 115, no. 2 (2016): 212–225. doi:10.1017/S0007114515004316.

McCartney, Margaret. "Margaret McCartney: Clean Eating and the Cult of Healthism." *British Medical Journal* 354, no. i4095 (2016). doi:10.1136/bmj.i4095.

McCarty, Mark F., and James J. Dinicolantonio. "Lauric Acid-rich Medium-chain Triglycerides Can Substitute for Other Oils in Cooking Applications and May Have Limited Pathogenicity." *Open Heart* 3, no. 2 (2016). doi:10.1136/openhrt-2016-000467.

McGuire, Shelley. "Scientific Report of the 2015 Dietary Guidelines Advisory Committee. Washington, DC: US Departments of Agriculture and Health and Human Services, 2015." *Advances in Nutrition* 7, no. 1 (2016): 202–204. doi:10.3945/an.115.011684.

McIntosh, Keith, David E. Reed, Theresa Schneider, et al. "FODMAPs Alter Symptoms and the Metabolome of Patients with IBS: A Randomised Controlled Trial." *Gut* 66, no. 7 (2016): 1241–1251. doi:10.1136/gutjnl-2015-311339.

Miquel-Kergoat, Sophie, Veronique Azais-Braesco, Britt Burton-Freeman, and Marion M. Hetherington. "Effects of Chewing on Appetite, Food Intake and Gut Hormones: A Systematic Review and Meta-analysis." *Physiology & Behavior* 151 (2015): 88–96. doi:10.1016/j.physbeh.2015.07.017.

Mukamal, Kenneth J., Catherine M. Clowry, Margaret M. Murray, et al. "Moderate Alcohol Consumption and Chronic Disease: The Case for a Long-Term Trial." *Alcoholism: Clinical and Experimental Research* 40, no. 11 (2016): 2283–2291. doi:10.1111/acer.13231.

National Institute of Diabetes and Digestive and Kidney Diseases. "Your Digestive System & How It Works." December 1, 2017. https://www.niddk.nih.gov/health-information/digestive-diseases/digestive-system-how-it-works.

Navarro, Victor J., Huiman Barnhart, Herbert L. Bonkovsky, et al. "Liver Injury from Herbals and Dietary Supplements in the US Drug-Induced Liver Injury Network." *Hepatology* 60, no. 4 (2014): 1399–1408. doi:10.1002/hep.27317.

Oken, Emily, Lauren B. Guthrie, Arienne Bloomingdale, et al. "A Pilot Randomized Controlled Trial to Promote Healthful Fish Consumption During Pregnancy: The Food for Thought Study." *Nutrition Journal* 12, no. 1 (2013). doi:10.1186/1475-2891-12-33.

Pimpin, Laura, Jason H. Y. Wu, Hila Haskelberg, Liana Del Gobbo, and Dariush Mozaffarian. "Is Butter Back? A Systematic Review and Meta-Analysis of Butter Consumption and Risk of Cardiovascular Disease, Diabetes, and Total Mortality." *Plos One* 11, no. 6 (2016). doi:10.1371/journal.pone.0158118.

Qian, Qi. "Dietary Influence on Body Fluid Acid-Base and Volume Balance: The Deleterious 'Norm' Furthers and Cloaks Subclinical Pathophysiology." *Nutrients* 10, no. 6 (2018): 778. doi:10.3390/nu10060778.

Rippe, James M., and Theodore J. Angelopoulos. "Sucrose, High-Fructose Corn Syrup, and Fructose, Their Metabolism and Potential Health Effects: What Do We Really Know?" *Advances in Nutrition* 4, no. 2 (2013): 236–245. doi:10.3945/an.112.002824.

Rodiño-Janeiro, B. K., M. Vicario, C. Alonso-Cotoner, R. Pascua-García, and J. Santos. "A Review of Microbiota and Irritable Bowel Syndrome: Future in Therapies." *Advances in Therapy* 35, no. 3 (2018): 289–310. doi:10.1007/s12325-018-0673-5.

Rubin, R. "Will Posting Nutritional Information on Menus Prod Diners to Make Healthier Choices?" *Journal of the American Medical Association* 319, no. 19 (2018): 1969–1971. doi:10.1001/jama.2018.3729.

Ruxton, C., S. Reed, M. Simpson, and K. Millington. "The Health Benefits of Omega-3 Polyunsaturated Fatty Acids: A Review of the Evidence." *Journal of Human Nutrition and Dietetics* 20, no. 3 (2007): 275–285. doi:10.1111/j.1365-277x.2007.00770.x.

Ryan, Meghan. "Daubert Standard." LII/Legal Information Institute. March 8, 2015. https://www.law.cornell.edu/wex/daubert_standard.

Sacks, F. M., A. H. Lichtenstein, J. H. Y. Wu, et al., on behalf of the American Heart Association. "Dietary Fats and Cardiovascular Disease: A Presidential Advisory from the American Heart Association." *Circulation* 136 (2017): e1–e23. doi: 10.1161/CIR.0000000000000510.

Savage, Jessica, and Christina B. Johns. Immunology and Allergy Clinics of North America. February 2015. Accessed June 1, 2018. https://www.ncbi.nlm.nih.gov/pmc/articles/PMC4254585/.

Schubert, Matthew M., Surendran Sabapathy, Michael Leveritt, and Ben Desbrow. "Acute Exercise and Hormones Related to Appetite Regulation: A Meta-Analysis." *Sports Medicine* 44, no. 3 (2013): 387–403. doi:10.1007/s40279-013-0120-3.

Smith, Andrea D., Alison Fildes, Lucy Cooke, Moritz Herle, Nicholas Shakeshaft, Robert Plomin, and Clare Llewellyn. "Genetic and Environmental Influences on Food Preferences in Adolescence." *American Journal of Clinical Nutrition* 104, no. 2 (2016): 446–453. doi:10.3945/ajcn.116.133983.

Sotos-Prieto, Mercedes, Shilpa N. Bhupathiraju, Josiemer Mattei, et al. "Association of Changes in Diet Quality with Total and Cause-Specific

Mortality." *New England Journal of Medicine* 377 (2017): 143–53. doi:10.1056/NEJMoa1613502.

Steele, Eurídice Martínez, Larissa Galastri Baraldi, Maria Laura Da Costa Louzada, Jean-Claude Moubarac, Dariush Mozaffarian, and Carlos Augusto Monteiro. "Ultra-Processed Foods and Added Sugars in the US Diet: Evidence from a Nationally Representative Cross-sectional Study." *BMJ Open* 6, no. 3 (2016). doi:10.1136/bmjopen-2015-009892.

Sueth-Santiago, Vitor, Gustavo Peron Mendes-Silva, Débora Decoté-Ricardo, and Marco Edilson Freire De Lima. "Curcumin, the Golden Powder from Turmeric: Insights into Chemical and Biological Activities." *Química Nova* (2015). doi:10.5935/0100-4042.20150035.

Sylvetsky, Allison C., and William H. Dietz. "Nutrient-Content Claims—Guidance or Cause for Confusion?" *New England Journal of Medicine* 371, no. 3 (2014): 195–198. doi:10.1056/nejmp1404899.

Tamanna, Nahid, and Niaz Mahmood. "Emerging Roles of Branched-Chain Amino Acid Supplementation in Human Diseases." *International Scholarly Research Notices* 2014 (2014): 1–8. doi:10.1155/2014/235619.

Tan, B. L., M. E. Norhaizan, and W-P-P Liew. "Nutrients and Oxidative Stress: Friend or Foe?" *Oxidative Medicine and Cellular Longevity* (2018): 9719584. doi:10.1155/2018/9719584.

Teigen, Karl Halvor. "Yerkes-Dodson: A Law for All Seasons." *Theory & Psychology* 4, no. 4 (1994): 525–547. doi:10.1177/0959354394044004.

Thorning, Tanja Kongerslev, Anne Raben, Tine Tholstrup, Sabita S. Soedamah-Muthu, Ian Givens, and Arne Astrup. "Milk and Dairy Products: Good or Bad for Human Health? An Assessment of the Totality of Scientific Evidence." *Food & Nutrition Research* 60, no. 1 (2016): 32527. doi:10.3402/fnr.v60.32527.

Thornton, Simon N. "Increased Hydration Can Be Associated with Weight Loss." *Frontiers in Nutrition* 3 (2016). doi:10.3389/fnut.2016.00018.

Tojo, R., A. Suárez, M. G. Clemente, et al. "Intestinal Microbiota in Health and Disease: Role of Bifidobacteria in Gut Homeostasis." *World Journal of Gastroenterology* 20, no. 41 (2014): 15163–15176. doi:10.3748/wjg.v20 .i41.15163.

Varady, Krista A. "Meal Frequency and Timing." *Current Opinion in Endocrinology & Diabetes and Obesity* 23, no. 5 (2016): 379–383. doi:10.1097/ med.0000000000000280.

Vaughn, Amber E., Chantel L. Martin, and Dianne S. Ward. "What Matters Most—What Parents Model or What Parents Eat?" *Appetite* 126 (2018): 102–107. doi.org/10.1016/j.appet.2018.03.025.

Wallace, Taylor C., and Victor L. Fulgoni. "Assessment of Total Choline Intakes in the United States." *Journal of the American College of Nutrition* 35, no. 2 (2016): 108–112. doi:10.1080/07315724.2015.1080127.

Wang, X., X. Lin, Y. Ouyang, et al. "Red and Processed Meat Consumption and Mortality: Dose-Response Meta-analysis of Prospective Cohort Studies." *Public Health Nutrition* 19, no. 5 (2016): 893–905. doi:10.1017/S1368980015002062.

Wang, X., Y. Ouyang, J. Liu, et al. "Fruit and Vegetable Consumption and Mortality from All Causes, Cardiovascular Disease, and Cancer: Systematic Review and Dose-Response Meta-analysis of Prospective Cohort Studies." *BMJ* 349, no. g4490 (2014). doi:10.1136/bmj.g4490.

White, John S. "Straight Talk about High-Fructose Corn Syrup: What It Is and What It Ain't." *American Journal of Clinical Nutrition* 88, no. 6 (2008). doi:10.3945/ajcn.2008.25825b.

Wu, Helen W., et al. "Changes in the Energy and Sodium Content of Main Entrées in US Chain Restaurants from 2010 to 2011." *Journal of the Academy of Nutrition and Dietetics* 114, no. 2: 209–219.

Wu, Yili, Long Zhai, and Dongfeng Zhang. "Sleep Duration and Obesity Among Adults: A Meta-analysis of Prospective Studies." *Sleep Medicine* 15, no. 12 (2014): 1456–1462. doi:10.1016/j.sleep.2014.07.018.

Wysoczański, Tomasz, Ewa Sokoła-Wysoczańska, Jolanta Pękala, et al. "Omega-3 Fatty Acids and Their Role in Central Nervous System—A Review." *Current Medicinal Chemistry* 23, no. 8 (2016): 816–831. doi:10.2174/0929867323666160122114439.

Zakim, David, and Thomas D. Boyer. *Hepatology: A Textbook of Liver Disease.* Saunders, 2003.

Zdzieblik, Denise, Steffen Oesser, Manfred W. Baumstark, Albert Gollhofer, and Daniel König. "Collagen Peptide Supplementation in Combination with Resistance Training Improves Body Composition and Increases Muscle Strength in Elderly Sarcopenic Men: A Randomised Controlled Trial." *British Journal of Nutrition* 114, no. 8 (2015): 1237–1245. doi:10.1017/s0007114515002810.

Zhang, Hua, and Rong Tsao. "Dietary Polyphenols, Oxidative Stress and Antioxidant and Anti-inflammatory Effects." *Current Opinion in Food Science* 8 (2016): 33–42. doi:10.1016/j.cofs.2016.02.002.

Zhang, Yuanting, Mark A. Kantor, and Wenyen Juan. "Usage and Understanding of Serving Size Information on Food Labels in the United States." *American Journal of Health Promotion* 30, no. 3 (2016): 181–87. doi:10.4278/ajhp.130117-quan-30.

Zion Market Research. "Global Dietary Supplements Market Will Reach USD 220.3 Billion in 2022: Zion Market Research." Globe Newswire News Room. January 11, 2017. https://globenewswire.com/news-release/2017/01/11/905073/0/en/Global-Dietary-Supplements-Market-will-reach-USD-220-3-Billion-in-2022-Zion-Market-Research.html.

Index

Page numbers of illustrations appear in italics.

About Jaclyn London

Jackie is a registered dietitian (RD) and New York State–Certified Dietitian-Nutritionist (CDN). As *Good Housekeeping*'s nutrition director, she is responsible for the creation, execution, and oversight of the brand's nutrition-related content across media platforms, and Good Housekeeping Seal applications in the food space. In 2016, she was responsible for the inception and strategic development of the Good Housekeeping Nutritionist Approved Emblem, a program that she continues to oversee and expand.

Jackie earned her bachelor's degree in history and dance from Northwestern University, and her master's degree in Clinical Nutrition and Dietetics from New York University. Before transitioning into magazine journalism in 2014, she served as senior clinical dietitian at the Mount Sinai Hospital, specializing in medical nutrition therapy for brain injury, stroke, and neurosurgical rehab. Additionally, Jackie counseled clients for weight-loss management, sports/athletics training, and other medical nutrition therapy interventions at the private practice Nutrition Energy in Manhattan. She's served as adjunct professor in biology at Touro College, and regularly participates in speaking engagements, presentations, and panels on behalf of *Good Housekeeping*.

To date, she's appeared on a number of national TV segments on behalf of the brand, including the *Today Show*, *The Rachael Ray Show*, *The Dr. Oz Show*, and *Inside Edition*, and appears regularly on local news outlets, including Fox5NY and *ABC News*.

Jackie was born and raised in New York, which is also where she currently resides.

Follow Jackie on Twitter/Instagram: @jaclynlondonrd.